PILATES
illustrated

Portia Page

Human Kinetics

Library of Congress Cataloging-in-Publication Data

Page, Portia, 1962-
 Pilates illustrated / Portia Page.
  p. cm.
 ISBN-13: 978-0-7360-9290-6 (soft cover)
 ISBN-10: 0-7360-9290-0 (soft cover)
 1. Pilates method. I. Title.
 RA781.4.P34 2011
 613.7'192--dc22

                          2010029436

ISBN-10: 0-7360-9290-0 (print)
ISBN-13: 978-0-7360-9290-6 (print)

This publication is written and published to provide accurate and authoritative information relevant to the subject matter presented. It is published and sold with the understanding that the author and publisher are not engaged in rendering legal, medical, or other professional services by reason of their authorship or publication of this work. If medical or other expert assistance is required, the services of a competent professional person should be sought.

Acquisitions Editor: Tom Heine; **Developmental Editor:** Cynthia McEntire; **Assistant Editor:** Elizabeth Evans; **Copyeditor:** Patricia L. MacDonald; **Graphic Designer:** Bob Reuther; **Graphic Artist:** Francine Hamerski; **Cover Designer:** Keith Blomberg; **Photographer (cover and interior):** Paul Body Photography; **Visual Production Assistant:** Joyce Brumfield; **Photo Production Manager:** Jason Allen; **Printer:** Courier Companies, Inc.

Human Kinetics books are available at special discounts for bulk purchase. Special editions or book excerpts can also be created to specification. For details, contact the Special Sales Manager at Human Kinetics.

Printed in the United States of America   10 9 8 7 6 5 4 3 2 1

The paper in this book is certified under a sustainable forestry program.

Human Kinetics
Web site: www.HumanKinetics.com

United States: Human Kinetics
P.O. Box 5076
Champaign, IL 61825-5076
800-747-4457
e-mail: humank@hkusa.com

Canada: Human Kinetics
475 Devonshire Road Unit 100
Windsor, ON N8Y 2L5
800-465-7301 (in Canada only)
e-mail: info@hkcanada.com

Europe: Human Kinetics
107 Bradford Road
Stanningley
Leeds LS28 6AT, United Kingdom
+44 (0) 113 255 5665
e-mail: hk@hkeurope.com

Australia: Human Kinetics
57A Price Avenue
Lower Mitcham, South Australia 5062
08 8372 0999
e-mail: info@hkaustralia.com

New Zealand: Human Kinetics
P.O. Box 80
Torrens Park, South Australia 5062
0800 222 062
e-mail: info@hknewzealand.com

E5133

PILATES
illustrated

Contents

Preface

I was first introduced to Pilates while competing in the National Aerobics Championship. My friend and mentor, Bruno Bosardi, introduced our team to Pilates, and I thought, *Okay, I'll give this a try. What can it hurt?* It was certainly better than throwing my body to the ground and landing in the splits or in a push-up, and it actually felt good. It felt positive and right, a very intuitive and beneficial form of exercise that would save my body from the wear and tear of the continual hard poundings and landings. Little did I know that I would soon become a Pilates instructor myself, much less a trainer of trainers.

What I found is that Pilates entered every aspect of my life. I soon realized that the principles of Pilates for better posture, a clear mind, and an efficient body enhanced my teaching of aerobics, cycling, kickboxing, and strength training. Pilates inspired me to become a better instructor, a better teacher, and a better mentor because the principles of Pilates matched what I had found to be innate in teaching. That first introduction has turned into a lifelong dream of teaching through intuition and a passion for what I am doing and giving to others. From the first Pilates workshop I led in Seoul, Korea, teaching a young group of personal trainers and group exercise instructors, I knew this was what I wanted to do and that I wanted to offer this to the world. Writing this book allowed me to do just that.

Approaching Pilates for the first time can be intimidating even to the most proficient fitness enthusiast, but with a little bit of understanding and time, the moves become intuitive and flow easily. The effects of a regular Pilates practice can be richly rewarding as well as relaxing or invigorating, depending on the style and pace at which you perform the exercises. Whether you are new to Pilates or just curious about it, *Pilates Illustrated* will give you a practical and hands-on guide to incorporating Pilates into your daily life.

In this book, you will find more than 100 individual exercises detailed and photographed as well as 17 Pilates workout programs to get you started. Exercises are listed in categories and defined by the starting body position. Photos of each exercise show the movement from beginning to end along with variations for modifications and challenges. For each exercise, the benefits, contraindications, breathing instructions, and alignment setup are listed. A step-by-step instruction list is given for each exercise as well as the focus and emphasis of each move.

Chapter 1 covers the benefits, history, and principles of Pilates, as well as the essential information on how to start your Pilates practice. The history of Pilates is relatively short but impressive. It is important to understand the major milestones in the development and evolution of Pilates. The physical and mental benefits of Pilates are discussed so you can understand the changes as they are occurring while you develop your practice of Pilates.

Starting your practice begins with learning how breath affects movement and how to breathe correctly so as to move with efficiency and ease. Mastering breathing can help in so many ways, from facilitating the move, to challenging your position, to providing a moment to pause and take in the benefits of the move.

Chapters 2 through 10 detail the more than 100 exercises in the book. Each exercise is accompanied by photos depicting the starting position, progression moves, and ending position. Included with the pictures is a comprehensive list of setup cues to get you into the correct position and follow-up cues to help you progress through the move to the final position. Exercises are classified by the starting position of the body: standing warm-up and stretch sequences; kneeling exercises; side-lying exercises; and prone, supine, and seated exercises. You will learn about the benefits of each move as well as the contraindications. Modifications for specific issues and challenges for more intermediate or advanced versions of each exercise are provided. Although the majority of exercises are mat focused, exercises that use small equipment such as a stability ball, Pilates ring, and stretch band are included. These pieces of equipment provide a different stimulus for the body and supplement your Pilates practice.

After the mat exercises, chapters 8, 9, and 10 feature Pilates exercises that use props—a stability ball, Pilates ring, and stretch band. Although Joseph Pilates didn't use stability balls or stretch bands (these are more recent developments in the Pilates world), these props, along with the Pilates ring, provide several benefits, from creating more or less stability to making an exercise more or less challenging. These props enhance and modify traditional Pilates exercises. In some cases, the prop will make the exercise more difficult by challenging the core or extremities or by increasing the intensity. In others, the prop makes the exercise more accessible to all levels of participants. The exercises for each prop are divided into standing or seated, side lying, prone, and supine. Each prop—the stability ball, Pilates ring, and stretch band—provides a diverse and different feel for the standard or modified Pilates moves described in earlier chapters. Standard safety guidelines and more advanced moves are included for each prop. These props are great tools for providing diversity and variety in your workouts as well as providing an avenue to progress to a more difficult exercise or series of movements.

Chapter 11 details 17 Pilates programs drawn from the individual exercises, including routines for weight loss, morning and evening workouts, the total body band, and advanced Pilates on the ball. They are in order based on the category or title name. These well-rounded workouts will satisfy practitioners at all levels and help you work around any time constraints you have. The time to complete a workout varies depending on your fitness level and the rate at which you complete the movement of each exercise. Everyone can find something in these routines. Included with these programs is the approximate time needed to complete the workout, the equipment needed, and the level of the workout so you can select the routine that works for you.

Keep in mind that you want to work with precision. Pay attention to each and every move your body makes, working methodically and slowly through each move to attain the desired results. Consistency is important; as Joseph H. Pilates said, "In 10 sessions, you will feel the difference. In 20, you will see the difference. And in 30, you'll be on your way to having a whole new body."

I've been fortunate to travel the world teaching Pilates and spreading the word about this fantastic form of exercise. In all of my travels, I have found that Pilates is appropriate for every population—young and old, male and female, athlete and nonathlete. No matter where you are, you can do Pilates and feel its profound effects and benefits. It is a language that everyone can speak and do and accomplish, whether you are in southern California; Shanghai, China; Bangkok, Thailand; the Czech Republic; or Saipan.

This book will guide everyone—from the first-time student to the Pilates enthusiast—to the true benefits of Pilates. Enjoy, and stand straight and tall!

Acknowledgments

Many people have contributed to this book in so many different ways. Thanks to Human Kinetics for asking me to write this book and providing me with the utmost patience and skill in getting through this process. Thanks to Bruno Bosardi for being my first Pilates mentor and Nora St. John for being a fearless director and leader as well as coach and friend. Thanks to Lizbeth Garcia and Judy King as my best friends forever (BFFs) as well as true role models whom I fully respect and admire. Thank you to the entire gang at Balanced Body for providing an outlet for my ideas and a platform to present them to the world. Thank you to Paul Body for being such a great photographer, and to the models in the book—Bruno Bosardi, Beth Pladson, and Lizbeth Garcia—for being so patient and so talented. Thanks to my family, especially my mom and aunts for their love and support and the wonderful womanly advice and care they have given me throughout the years, as well as their undying belief in me, and my brother and his wife and kids for always making me smile and to remember the simple things in life. Thanks to my clients and students over the years who constantly remind me that I have the greatest job in the world!

A special thank you to my wonderful boyfriend and partner Gary Huhn and our dog, Nestle, for their devotion and faith, for putting up with me over the last year with the all-nighters and weekends devoted to writing and missing out on the family outings, and for lifting my spirits and putting a smile on my face when I didn't think I could go on. Also, my efforts are in honor of my grandmother, Corinne Ellen Walaity, who always reminded me that, as stated by William Earnest Henley in *Invictus*, "I am the master of my fate; I am the captain of my soul."

Chapter 1

Art and Practice of Pilates

Pilates is something you can do a little of every day with amazing results. It is an exercise designed to elongate and strengthen the body by emphasizing balance, alignment, proper breathing, and core stability and strength. Joseph H. Pilates understood that a healthy body leads to a healthy mind: "Physical fitness is the first requisite of happiness." After a few sessions of Pilates, you too can understand how helpful correct and flowing movement can be to your mind and body.

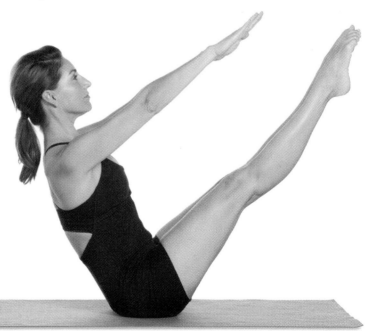

Benefits of Pilates

The benefits of Pilates (called *contrology* by Joseph Pilates) are summed up nicely in this quote from its creator: "Contrology develops the body uniformly, corrects wrong postures, restores physical vitality, invigorates the mind, and elevates the spirit."

Pilates, now a household name, can help you stand taller and move and look better in a relatively short time. Anyone at any age and with almost any condition can perform the exercises easily. Pilates is practiced in homes, studios, fitness centers, and rehabilitation clinics worldwide to help people rehabilitate from injuries, increase flexibility and strength, and improve their overall health and wellness. There are numerous benefits to doing Pilates, but these are the most common ones:

- ▶ Creates body awareness
- ▶ Develops long and strong muscles
- ▶ Leads to easier and more agile movements
- ▶ Increases flexibility
- ▶ Strengthens the entire core
- ▶ Improves overall posture

These six benefits go a long way to developing a more fit and active body as well as a deeper connection with the mind and spirit.

With a regular Pilates practice, the use of precision with every movement helps create an acute awareness of your own body. This is critical to attaining the most from your workout. Once you have developed body awareness, you can begin to build strength. This strength is gained in long and lean musculature that is not bulky or restrictive. Once the muscles are moving in unison and with length and strength, all of your body's movements, small and large, will be more graceful, easier to perform, and more efficient.

Pilates also increases overall flexibility of the body and limbs. This in turn helps with ease of movement and also will improve movement and decrease tightness in areas such as the back, hips, and shoulders. Core strengthening is one of the biggest goals and benefits in Pilates as everything is generated and conducted from the center, or powerhouse, of the body. If one has a strong powerhouse, then strong limbs and organs naturally develop.

Good posture is one of the most noticeable benefits of Pilates and can be attained in the first session. A small difference in posture—moving the head and neck slightly back and up, rolling back the shoulders, lifting the rib cage off the hips—can make a huge difference in a person's outside appearance and in the way he or she moves. The most common thing people say after their first Pilates session, or even their 10th or 20th, is that they feel better. They not only feel better but also move better and look better. The key noticeable improvement is posture. When you stand taller and straighter, you feel better and move with more ease. Good posture can help alleviate some back pain almost immediately, and this is what I think is so wonderful about Pilates.

History of Pilates

Joseph Pilates urged people to realize the importance and benefits of a perfectly balanced body and mind and preached that his exercise regimen, which he called *contrology*, would do just that. He believed that to achieve the most within our capabilities we have to constantly strive to acquire strong, healthy bodies and develop our minds to the limits of our ability. Although this concept and the more recent publicity about the mind–body connection and Pilates have become increasingly popular in the last decade, it is amazing to think that he developed contrology in the early 1900s.

A man far ahead of his time, he was in incredible shape even into his mid-80s and followed his own exercise routine to maintain his strength and flexibility until his death in 1967. Born in the late 1800s in Germany, Joseph Pilates suffered from several childhood diseases (asthma, rheumatic fever, and rickets) that left him with a weak respiratory system. He spent his life overcoming his frailties and developing his workout regimen; he became an accomplished athlete and physical specimen, even posing for anatomical drawings at age 14. During the early 1900s, a new awareness of health that was centered on exercise began to spring up. Revelations about the positive effects of exercise on the mind and body were in the making, and Joseph Pilates was right in the forefront of all this. The influences of these new ideas as well as the change in his own body enabled him to develop contrology.

During World War I, Pilates was interned in a camp in England and after the war returned to Germany for a short while before immigrating to the United States in 1926. On the way over to the United States, he met his wife, Clara, and they settled in New York City, where he opened his studio on 8th Avenue, attracting many dancers, athletes, and businessmen. Since his studio was located in the same building as the New York City Ballet, he worked with many dancers and had huge success with healing and helping injured dancers; thus his work became very popular with the dance community. Even so, he envisioned his work being done by anyone and everyone, from schoolchildren to housewives to business executives.

Although his work was not acknowledged much in his lifetime, a few of the people he taught went on to continue his work and in the last 20 years have brought Pilates into the mainstream of exercise. Some of those who worked with Joseph Pilates are Romana Kryzanowska, Ron Fletcher, Kathleen Stanford Grant, Lolita San Miguel, and Mary Bowen, many of whom still teach today. Today, some 10 million people in the United States alone use Pilates as their method of exercise (*Pilates Style*, January 2009). Although Pilates was developed in the early 1900s, it's taken some time to develop into the phenomenon it is today. The popularity has grown as the benefits have come to light, with people getting results and feeling better. Word of mouth, as well as key people in the media touting its benefits, has made Pilates widespread in gyms, studios, and homes throughout the world.

Joseph Pilates created an effective combination of stretching and strengthening that works for practically every body. His greatest legacy remains his classic mat exercises, the original 34 exercises detailed in his book *Return to Life Through Contrology*. Many Pilates schools teach or progress the exercises differently, with the end product being an evolving method. Although some of the more recent fitness research might suggest that his ideas of spinal alignment are not ideal and that you need to use caution when performing some of the exercises, especially if you have certain conditions or pain, for the most part his original ideas and exercises are still sound and will help create a practical solution to fix posture and alignment issues. In this book, I have chosen to use most of the original 34 exercises (although in a different order) as a base and have developed modifications and transitions and exercises that make the flow more achievable or more challenging. The use of props is also an addition and is not considered classical, but it allows a way to expand on the original exercises.

In 1965, at the age of 86, Joseph Pilates said, "I must be right. Never an Aspirin. Never injured a day in my life. The whole country, the whole world, should be doing my exercises. They'd be happier." Some food for thought!

Pilates Principles

Pilates is a method of exercise that connects the mind and the body as one and allows the body to move in a more efficient way. This form of exercise uses your body to its greatest advantage, utilizing your own strength, flexibility, and coordination, and requires that you pay attention to your body throughout each movement. To help achieve this powerful mind–body connection, the following six principles should be kept in mind.

▶ **Breathing.** Controlling the breath and breathing correctly are extremely important to understanding Pilates and obtaining the fullest benefits from the exercise. Breathing properly is the first thing you should focus on, and you should maintain this focus throughout the movement. Focused, controlled breathing will help you maintain proper alignment as well as allow you to contract the muscles that need to be contracted and release those that don't need to be used. Breathing fully and correctly will also help with the flow of the exercise and movements and allow you to continue a program all the way through. Breathing brings in oxygen to your system and clears the head, thus facilitating movement.

▶ **Concentration.** This involves the important connection between the mind and the body. Paying attention to what you are doing is critical for moving correctly and easily. Concentration allows the mind to control and move the body efficiently and appropriately.

▶ **Control.** Each movement in Pilates is controlled and should never be wasted. Keeping the movement within your capabilities is important for maintaining alignment and stability throughout the body during the exercises.

▶ **Centering.** Everything in Pilates is initiated from the center of the body, called the powerhouse or core. To perform the movements correctly, begin from the center. Building a strong, stable, and flexible center is one of the best outcomes of doing Pilates on a regular basis. A strong center makes for a strong body overall.

▶ **Precision.** Practicing concentration, control, and centering will make each movement precise and totally correct. Be conscious and aware of every part of your body, and continually check your alignment and form to ensure that you are performing each exercise with precision.

▶ **Flowing movement or rhythm.** Having all your muscles working together with precision from your center and with concentration and control as well as correct breathing creates a rhythmic and flowing movement pattern. This means you are moving with extreme efficiency and flow and with just the right amount of effort. Be patient with yourself. Allow yourself the time needed for your body and mind to work together to produce flowing movement.

Lateral Breathing

The importance of breathing and the fact that we do it without thinking is summed up in this quote from Joseph Pilates: "Breathing is the first act of life, and the last." Even so, simply knowing that you are breathing is not enough. Breathing correctly and fully will make all the difference in your Pilates practice. Pilates exercises require you to breathe fully and deeply, using every inhale to take in lots of fresh air and every exhale to get rid of stale air. This process oxygenates the blood and gets the circulation going. Breathing fully and deeply can energize your every move. Breath is the very foundation of Pilates movement, and the exercises in this book are outlined with specific breathing instructions that coordinate with specific movements. The breath will be used to initiate and support movements as well as facilitate and energize the movements.

The breathing technique to use is called *lateral breathing*. Lateral breathing means breathing deeply and fully into the sides and back, or the lower lobes of the lungs. With this type of breath, you can keep the abdominal muscles contracted, providing support for the lower spine and back. To make this process smoother, inhale through the nose and exhale through the mouth, as if you were blowing out a candle. As you inhale through the nose, imagine your rib cage expanding out to the sides like an umbrella opening or an accordion playing. As you exhale through the mouth, imagine the rib cage drawing inward like a corset being tightened, bringing the rib cage toward the hip bones.

Proper lateral breathing is critical for achieving the correct alignment and focus in your Pilates practice. You might want to practice this type of breathing every day in front of a mirror so you can note the rib cage moving outward on the inhale and inward on the exhale, thereby making the actual exercises easier to follow and execute.

Pelvic Floor Engagement

What is the pelvic floor and why do you need to know how to engage it? Pilates instructors are often asked this question as this is a common mystery to most beginners. The pelvic floor is the support structure for the bladder, rectum, uterus in women, and prostate in men. The pelvic floor is the bottom layer of the deepest core musculature and the lower support of the abdominal cavity. It helps you breath and provides support for the spine.

Contraction of the deep pelvic floor muscles will help you engage the transversus abdominis, the natural girdle that lies roughly between the belly button and the pubic bone and wraps around the waist. The transversus abdominis is an important stabilizer for the lower back and the spine. Contracting the pelvic floor not only provides support it also aids in Pilates practice and improves posture in general.

Think of the pelvic floor as a hammock made of muscle that lies between the sit bones and the pubic bone and between the thighs. To engage this group of muscles, inhale and then as you exhale try to lift and tighten the pelvic floor. It should feel as if you are trying to stop the flow of urine or as if it were an elevator floor moving up. Try to not use any other muscles, such as the buttocks or abdominals, in this process. The movement will be small and mostly internal, unseen by others. Engaging the pelvic floor is something you can practice anytime during the day. As you practice, it should start to feel easy and automatic as you breathe.

Proper Alignment

Once you have mastered breathing and pelvic floor engagement, you must master the alignment of your spine and body in general. Ideally, working with a certified Pilates trainer in a studio will ensure that you are doing the exercises correctly and in the correct alignment. If this is not a possibility, try the following procedure in front of a mirror. You will use the most prominent markers on your body, the ones that are easy to see, to figure out your ideal alignment (figure 1.1). It is important to note that the only way to achieve good dynamic posture is through practice. Work at the following every day to achieve a good posture and starting point for the exercises. Starting from bottom to top, try to line up your body accordingly:

1. Stand in front of a full-length mirror looking straight on.

2. Start by looking at your legs; look down the legs and see if they line up evenly. You want to see the middle of the kneecap in line with the hip bone and the middle of the ankle joint under the middle of the knee.

3. Next look at your hips and see if the tops of your hips line up evenly. If not, try to level them as best as you can.

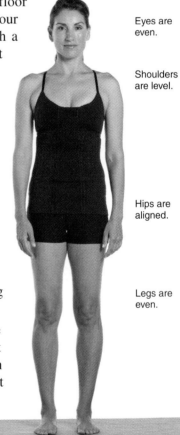

Eyes are even.

Shoulders are level.

Hips are aligned.

Legs are even.

Figure 1.1 Finding good standing alignment.

4. Next look at the level of your shoulders. Most people have one side that hikes up, creating stress in the upper back and neck area. Level your shoulders as best as you can without placing any stress on other parts of the body. This will become easier once you are warmed up, but do try to gain the correct alignment while standing in front of the mirror so you know what you need to try to attain while exercising.

5. Finish with your head. Look at your eyes and see if they line up. If they don't, your head might be tilting to one side, indicating a tightness in the torso or neck area. Try to level your eyes if they are not by making minute changes until your eyes look even and steady.

These adjustments might seem difficult or unattainable now, but at least note the alignment of your body in this position. Here you have a decent view of the front of your body without having to contort your body to see the side or back. It is best to see this alignment and be aware of it now, and then you can use this knowledge during your workout to chart your progress as you exercise.

For positions other than standing, learn the following criteria to align particular parts of the body (figures 1.2, 1.3, and 1.4). Keep in mind that muscular tightness or injuries can make the ideal alignment difficult to attain at first. Be patient. Work slowly within your range of motion, finding a way that allows minimal discomfort or pain.

Head position. When standing or sitting, the earlobes should be over the top line of the shoulders, with a slight inward curve of the spine at the cervical area. When lying on your back, relax the shoulders, and without force, allow the chin to drop in toward the chest as you feel a lengthening of the back of the neck. It might be necessary to place a small pillow or bath towel under the head for support. When kneeling, imagine your eyes looking straight ahead and the back of the neck lining up with a wall behind you. When on your abdomen, bring the forehead to the mat below you, again feeling the length in the back of the neck.

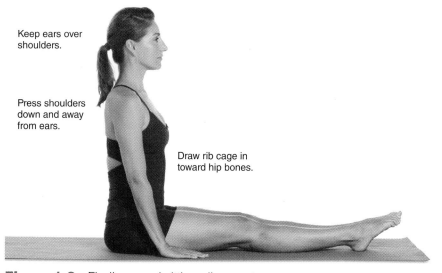

Keep ears over shoulders.

Press shoulders down and away from ears.

Draw rib cage in toward hip bones.

Figure 1.2 Finding good sitting alignment.

Lengthen the neck.

Make sure ASIS and public symphysis are parallel to floor.

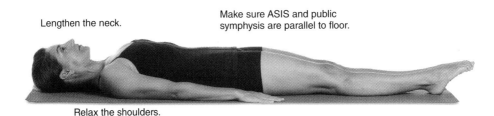

Relax the shoulders.

Figure 1.3   Finding good lying alignment.

Look straight head.

Keep the neck straight.

Press shoulders down and away from ears.

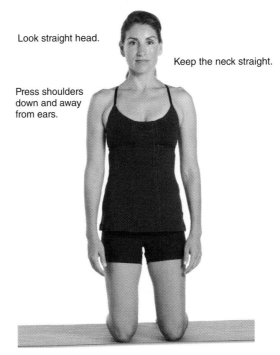

Figure 1.4   Finding good kneeling alignment.

Pelvic and spinal alignment. The neutral position of this area is defined when the ASIS (anterior superior iliac spine) and the pubic symphysis lie parallel to whatever plane you are lying in. For example, if you are lying on your back, they are parallel to the floor. If you are lying on your side, sitting, or kneeling, they are parallel to the wall in front of or behind you.

Rib cage position. When standing, sitting, or lying, draw the rib cage, especially the lower ribs, in toward the hip bones. Consider this a softening of this area, and work toward lengthening the back side of the body.

Scapula and shoulder position. The scapulae are the wings on your back. Basically they should glide evenly over the back of your rib cage. The shoulders should always ride down and away from the ears. Excessive rounding of the shoulders due to poor posture and sitting habits can make this position difficult to reach at first, but it is attainable over time if you are persistent and consistent with your practice.

When to Practice

Joseph Pilates recommended his exercises every day for just 15 minutes, and although Pilates is an exercise that you can do every day, this might not be realistic for your schedule.

It is important to set a practical exercise schedule that you can maintain rather than set a target of exercising every day and then not doing it. Accomplishment is a great motivator, and setting realistic goals is vital to that success. The breathing method discussed earlier can be practiced every day and is a great way to start or end your day. From there, try to set aside 10 to 15 minutes two times a week to attempt some of the beginning exercises. Once you have mastered these, try adding a few more and exercising for 20 to 30 minutes twice a week. If you are used to exercising, you might want to try a more rigorous workout from the routines in the last chapter or move onto the intermediate and advanced moves and increase your workout time to 45 to 60 minutes twice a week. From there, you can add more days or increase difficulty level or a little bit of both. Pilates is a nonimpact workout and can be done daily for remarkable results. Have fun with the routines, and note your level of flexibility and strength with each exercise so you can chart your progress.

Pilates is the perfect way to start exercising or to add to your current workout schedule. The results will come fast if you are loyal to your commitment!

When and What to Eat

Although there is no special eating regimen for Pilates, you should consider what foods, how much, and when to eat as you move toward a Pilates workout. To fully take advantage of Pilates as a mind–body workout, eat foods that keep you alert and balanced. Also, since Pilates exercises emphasize using the core, especially the abdominals, you will not want to be full. In fact, you probably will work better on a fairly empty stomach, although you do not want to run out of steam halfway through your workout. Complex carbohydrate and lean protein with a little high-quality fat are good choices as these will sustain energy better than simple carbohydrate or sugar. With Pilates, you do not necessarily need special sports drinks, but you will want to stay hydrated. Water is always an appropriate choice.

Safety

Before beginning an exercise chapter, review correct body alignment for your body type as it pertains to the exercises in that chapter. Please use caution when performing any exercise, especially if it is the first time you are doing it. If you have any injuries or chronic conditions or are pregnant, please see a doctor and get advice or clearance to exercise before beginning. The first few sessions of any new exercise program will be challenging as you figure out how to move and breathe. Be patient with yourself. Take the time to read through the directions, and practice each move several times. Once you have done them a few times, it will get easier and you will be able to move from exercise to exercise with better ease. Practice does make perfect!

Have fun!

Chapter 2

Standing Warm-Up Exercises and Stretches

The standing warm-up exercises and stretch sequences in this chapter lay the foundation for the remainder of the exercises by readying your mind and body for the various positions required for mat work. Learning to position your body in the correct alignment while standing is also fundamentally important to your everyday posture and overall balance. These exercises lay the basis for a solid Pilates practice by leaving you feeling awake, alive, and mobile as well as strong and stable.

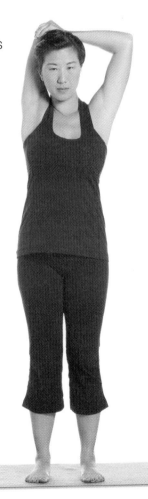

Modified Pilates Stance

Level
▶ Beginner

Contraindications
▶ Injuries to the lower back, hip, knee, ankle, or foot

Focus
▶ Entire body awareness and alignment

Benefits
▶ Develops awareness of the entire body
▶ Helps you find neutral or natural stance and correct alignment
▶ Focuses the mind and the body

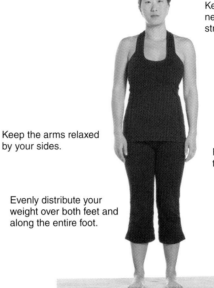

Reach the top of the head toward the ceiling.

Keep the back of the neck long and eyes straight ahead.

Keep the arms relaxed by your sides.

Reach the tailbone toward the floor.

Evenly distribute your weight over both feet and along the entire foot.

1 Place the feet in parallel position, like the number 11, with the heels underneath the sit bones. Inhale and feel the rib cage lift off the hips and lengthen the spine. Exhale and feel the rib cage draw in and back as the spine lengthens, long and tall. This is the standard start position for most standing exercises.

2 Take four or five breaths in this position. Begin to feel the tallness of the body. Each breath will help to center and focus your awareness on your entire body.

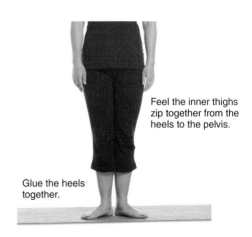

Feel the inner thighs zip together from the heels to the pelvis.

Variation
Inhale. Place the heels together. As you exhale, turn the toes out to form a little V with your feet.

Glue the heels together.

Shoulder Warming

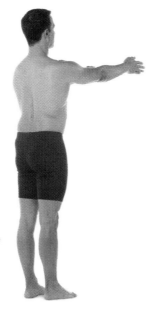

Level
▶ Beginner

Contraindications
▶ Injuries to the shoulder

Focus
▶ Muscles of the shoulder and upper back

Benefits
▶ Increases range of motion of scapula over the rib cage
▶ Promotes better posture and breathing
▶ Warms up and activates the shoulder girdle

1 Stand tall in modified Pilates stance with arms at shoulder height, palms turned in. Inhale and prepare the upper body for movement by engaging the abdominals and lengthening the spine.

2 Exhale and round shoulders forward, letting the scapulae separate wide. Allow the shoulders to glide forward toward fingertips. Hold the lower body steady. It should not move as the upper body moves with the breathing.

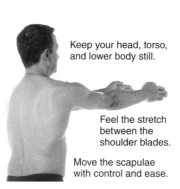

Keep your head, torso, and lower body still.

Feel the stretch between the shoulder blades.

Move the scapulae with control and ease.

3 Inhale. Squeeze shoulder blades past neutral and toward one another. Arms stay in front of shoulders. Each breath should allow you to move a bit deeper and feel the stretch a bit more. Repeat for 5 to 10 repetitions.

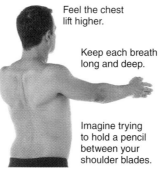

Feel the chest lift higher.

Keep each breath long and deep.

Imagine trying to hold a pencil between your shoulder blades.

Heel Raise With Squat

Level
▶ Beginner

Contraindications
▶ Injuries to the hip, knee, or ankle

Focus
▶ Legs
▶ Core

Benefits
▶ Warms up the body
▶ Builds coordination with breath and movement
▶ Prepares the body for more strenuous activity

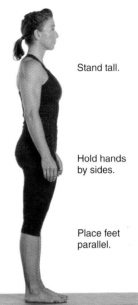

Stand tall.

Hold hands by sides.

Place feet parallel.

1 **Stand tall in a modified Pilates stance with a neutral pelvis, arms at sides, feet parallel. Achieve a neutral pelvis by bringing the hip bones (ASIS) and the pubic bone in a parallel triangle to the wall behind you. There should be no strain in the lower back muscles or hip flexors.**

Center weight over entire foot.

Keep shoulders down as arms lift overhead.

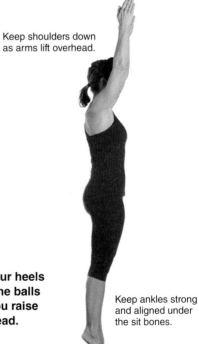

2 **Inhale. Lift your heels and balance on the balls of your feet as you raise your arms overhead.**

Keep ankles strong and aligned under the sit bones.

Gentle Variation
Lift heels only slightly off the mat or not at all.

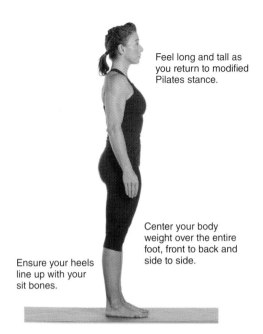

Feel long and tall as you return to modified Pilates stance.

Center your body weight over the entire foot, front to back and side to side.

Ensure your heels line up with your sit bones.

3 Exhale. Return to modified Pilates stance, arms by your sides.

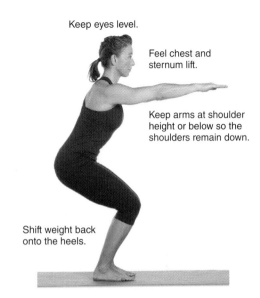

Keep eyes level.

Feel chest and sternum lift.

Keep arms at shoulder height or below so the shoulders remain down.

Shift weight back onto the heels.

4 Inhale. Bend the knees and press the hips back by hinging at the hips into a small squat. Bring the arms up to shoulder height as you squat back on both heels.

Gentle Variation
Keep knees straight as arms rise up to shoulder height.

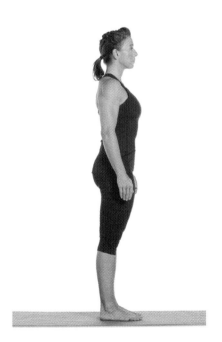

5 Exhale. Return to modified Pilates stance. Repeat for 5 to 10 repetitions.

Arm Stretch

Level

▶ Beginner

Contraindications

▶ Injuries to the lower back, shoulders, or arms

Focus

▶ Muscles of the upper arms, back, and shoulders

Benefits

▶ Warms up the upper body and arms
▶ Loosens the shoulder joints
▶ Allows the scapulae to slide freely for an increased range of motion
▶ Prepares the arms for bracing the upper body

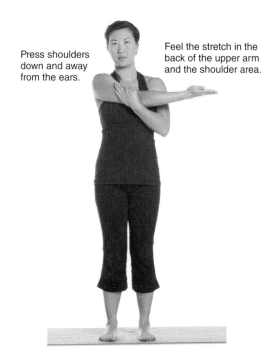

Press shoulders down and away from the ears.

Feel the stretch in the back of the upper arm and the shoulder area.

1 Stand tall. Cross the right arm over the body at chest height. Hold the right arm with the left hand above the right elbow. Press your shoulders down and away from your ears as if sliding the scapulae into your back pockets. Hold this stretch for 30 to 45 seconds or three or four breaths, and then repeat with the left arm.

2 Stand tall. Bring the right arm over the right shoulder, reaching the right hand behind the mid-back or near the left shoulder, depending on flexibility. The left hand holds the right elbow for a triceps stretch. You will feel the stretch from your right hip all the way up the side of your body and into the back of your upper arm. Hold this stretch for 30 to 45 seconds or three or four breaths, and then repeat with the left arm.

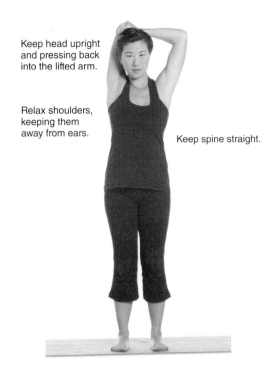

Keep head upright and pressing back into the lifted arm.

Relax shoulders, keeping them away from ears.

Keep spine straight.

3 Stand tall. Bring the right arm overhead and lean to the left. The left arm remains down by your side. This stretch helps open the intercostals (the muscles between the ribs), which will assist your breathing and let you take deeper breaths. Hold this stretch for 30 to 45 seconds or three or four breaths, and then repeat with the left arm.

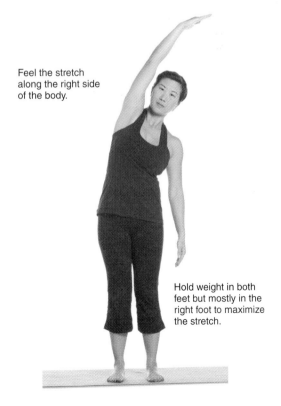

Feel the stretch along the right side of the body.

Hold weight in both feet but mostly in the right foot to maximize the stretch.

Leg Stretch

Level
▶ Beginner

Contraindications
▶ Injuries to the hips, knees, or ankles
▶ Vertigo

Focus
▶ Stretches for the legs, hips, and lower back

Benefits
▶ Warms up and loosens the legs and hips
▶ Develops balance and body control
▶ Prepares the lower body for more strenuous activity

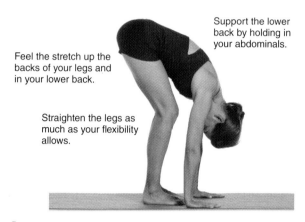

Feel the stretch up the backs of your legs and in your lower back.

Support the lower back by holding in your abdominals.

Straighten the legs as much as your flexibility allows.

1 Stand in modified Pilates stance. Inhale and fold the body forward as you bend your knees. Exhale and continue to roll down, bending more in the knees as needed. Allow the chest to come onto the thighs as you relax the shoulders. Hold the stretch for 30 to 45 seconds or three or four breaths, and then roll up to return to standing.

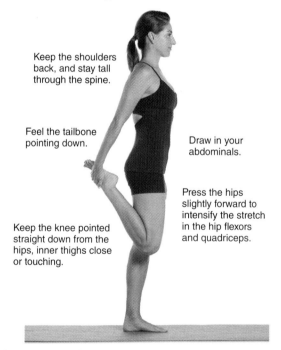

Keep the shoulders back, and stay tall through the spine.

Feel the tailbone pointing down.

Draw in your abdominals.

Keep the knee pointed straight down from the hips, inner thighs close or touching.

Press the hips slightly forward to intensify the stretch in the hip flexors and quadriceps.

2 Stand on your left leg. With your right hand, bring the right foot to the buttocks as the hips slide forward. Exhale as you press the foot into the hand, and feel the stretch in the hip flexors and quadriceps. Hold the stretch for 30 to 45 seconds or three or four breaths, and then switch legs.

3 Stand on the left leg, and cross the right ankle over the left thigh as you sit back into a mini-squat. Hands can stay at the hips or hang beside the body. Draw the abdominals in and up as you squat deeper to further stretch the lateral rotators. Hold the stretch for 30 to 45 seconds or three or four breaths, and then switch legs.

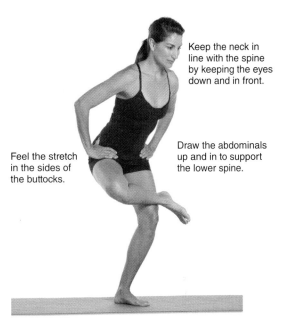

Keep the neck in line with the spine by keeping the eyes down and in front.

Draw the abdominals up and in to support the lower spine.

Feel the stretch in the sides of the buttocks.

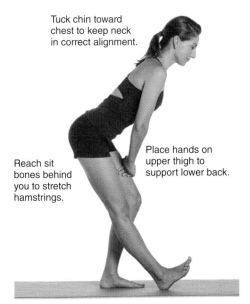

Tuck chin toward chest to keep neck in correct alignment.

Reach sit bones behind you to stretch hamstrings.

Place hands on upper thigh to support lower back.

Gentle Standing Variation

From modified Pilates stance, inhale and move your right leg slightly in front of you as you bend your left knee. Exhale as you hinge at the hips, bringing the upper body forward and down slightly. Place both hands on the left thigh to support the lower back. Hold the stretch for 30 to 45 seconds or three or four breaths. Switch legs.

Gentle Seated Variation

Sit with your right leg straight in front of and in line with your right hip. The left knee is bent with the foot coming in toward the right leg. Hinge at the hips to stretch the upper body forward. Exhale as you reach the sit bones behind you. Try to keep the spine straight and long and the shoulders pulling down and back as you reach forward toward the thigh or shin with both hands. Hold the stretch for 30 to 45 seconds or three or four breaths, and then switch legs.

Keep the neck in alignment with the spine by bringing the eyes down and front.

Support your lower back with your hands at the upper right thigh or shin.

Keep the sit bones reaching behind to stretch the hamstrings.

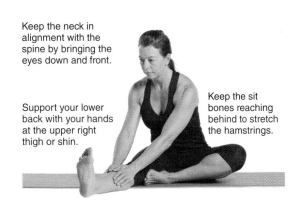

Pelvic Clock

Level
- Beginner

Contraindications
- Injuries to or chronic conditions of the spine

Focus
- Muscles of the trunk and pelvis

Benefits
- Creates awareness of and helps develop spinal articulation
- Increases flexibility in the lower back
- Warms up the spinal muscles
- Teaches the correct placement of the pelvis, neutral and centered

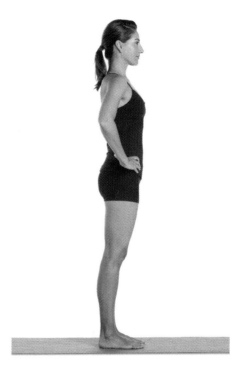

1 Stand tall in a modified Pilates stance with the hands at the hips. The hands at the hips will provide a great guideline for where and how the hips and pelvis are moving.

2 Begin the movement by engaging the pelvic floor and transverse abdominal muscles, as if your belly were being scooped out. Inhale as the tailbone lifts and the pelvis rocks into a slight arch (anterior tilt, or lordosis). This is the 6 o'clock position.

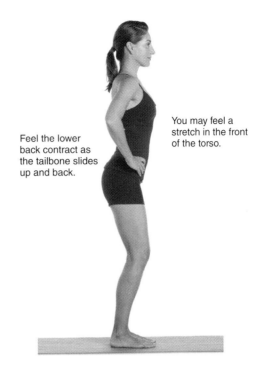

Feel the lower back contract as the tailbone slides up and back.

You may feel a stretch in the front of the torso.

3 Exhale as the abdominals scoop inward and the tailbone tucks under (posterior tilt). This is the 12 o'clock position. Repeat for 5 to 10 repetitions.

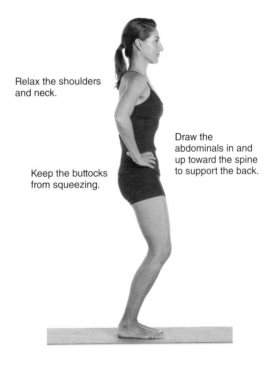

Relax the shoulders and neck.

Keep the buttocks from squeezing.

Draw the abdominals in and up toward the spine to support the back.

Roll-Down

Level
▶ Beginner

Contraindications
▶ Low or high blood pressure
▶ Injuries to or chronic conditions of the spine

Focus
▶ Muscles of the trunk and legs

Benefits
▶ Stretches the upper back and lower spine
▶ Stretches the hamstrings
▶ Develops and deepens spinal articulation

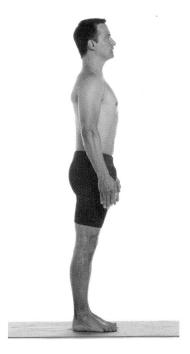

1 Stand tall in modified Pilates stance.

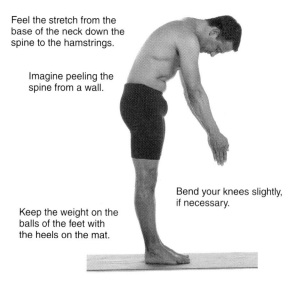

Feel the stretch from the base of the neck down the spine to the hamstrings.

Imagine peeling the spine from a wall.

Bend your knees slightly, if necessary.

Keep the weight on the balls of the feet with the heels on the mat.

2 Inhale as the chin lowers toward the chest. Roll down one vertebra at a time. Exhale as you continue to roll down and reach for the mat with your hands.

3 The upper body hangs over the floor, with the hands grazing or nearly touching the mat, depending on flexibility. Inhale and begin to roll up. Exhale as you continue to roll up until you are standing tall again. Imagine stacking the spine one vertebra at a time as you return to standing.

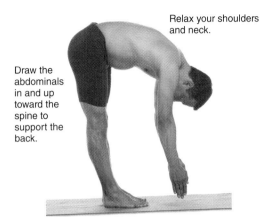

Relax your shoulders and neck.

Draw the abdominals in and up toward the spine to support the back.

Gentle Variation

If the hamstrings are tight, stop the roll-down with your forearms at your thighs and the knees bent. Round at the lower spine to stretch the spine. Tuck your chin toward your chest to keep the neck in correct alignment with the spine. Take a full breath, and roll back up to a standing upright position.

Keep the abdominals engaged to further support the lower spine

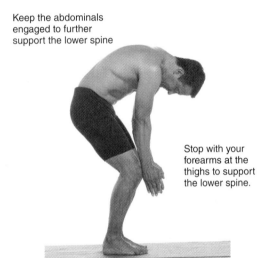

Stop with your forearms at the thighs to support the lower spine.

Shoulder Shrug

Level
- Beginner

Contraindications
- Injuries to the shoulder

Focus
- Muscles of the upper back and shoulders

Benefits
- Warms up the shoulder girdle
- Increases range of motion in the shoulder and scapula areas
- Prepares the upper body for more strenuous activity

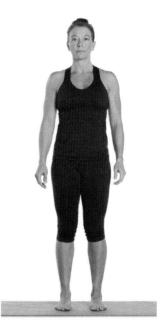

1 **Stand tall in modified Pilates stance with arms at sides, neutral pelvis and spine.**

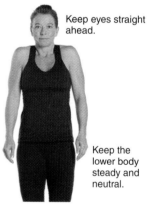

Keep eyes straight ahead.

2 **Inhale. Lift your shoulders toward your ears as if you were shrugging your shoulders. Feel the shoulders try to touch the ears like earrings.**

Keep the lower body steady and neutral.

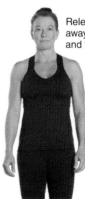

Release shoulders away from ears and toward floor.

3 **Exhale as you allow your shoulders to fall with a big release. Use gravity and momentum to release the shoulders down. The heavier the fall of the shoulders, the stronger the release in the upper body. Repeat for 5 to 10 repetitions.**

Move through the upper body with control and ease.

Keep your torso steady.

Chapter 3

Kneeling Mat Exercises

The kneeling exercises are a great way to continue to prepare for the lying mat exercises presented in the next chapter. Kneeling exercises warm up and prepare the body for more difficult work ahead, as well as allow the body to gain more mobility and flexibility. These exercises can be done on their own or as a warm-up or transition into the other exercises. The kneeling mat exercises are done on one knee and one hand, on both knees, or on hands and knees.

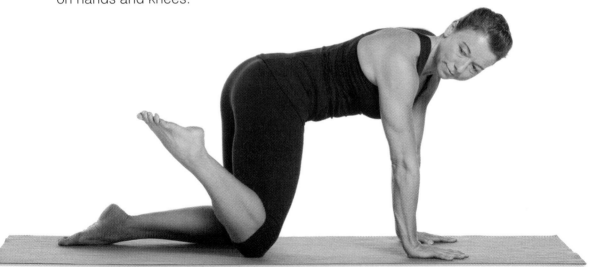

Child's Pose

Level
- Beginner

Contraindications
- Injuries to the knees, lower back, or shoulders

Focus
- Muscles of the back and shoulders

Benefits
- Stretches the entire back from the neck to the tailbone
- Creates mobility and range of motion in the shoulders
- Mobilizes the upper back
- Rests the wrists after kneeling or plank work

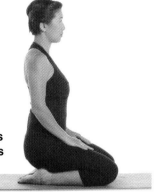

1 Sit on your heels with your big toes touching and the knees hip-distance apart or a bit wider. The tops of the feet are on the mat. Shoulders are over your hips, with hands resting on your thighs.

Keep abdominals drawing up and in to provide support for the lower spine.

Lengthen the spine from the head to the tailbone.

Relax your arms, and spread the fingertips wide.

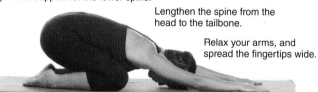

2 Lean forward and place your hands in front of your shoulders with straight arms. Bring your forehead to the mat in front of your knees. Hold this position for four to six breaths.

Gentle Variation 1
If the tops of your feet are really tight, you can tuck your toes under. If the tops of your thighs are extremely tight, increase the distance between your knees.

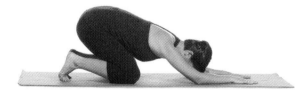

Gentle Variation 2
An option if you have tight shoulders or injuries is to make fists and stack one fist on top of the other, placing the forehead on the fists.

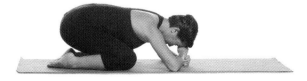

External Rotation With Arms

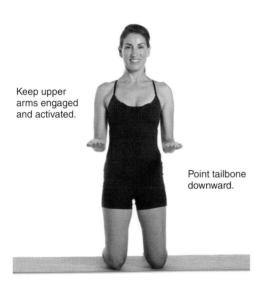

Keep upper arms engaged and activated.

Point tailbone downward.

Level
- ▶ Beginner

Contraindications
- ▶ Injuries to the lower back, spine, or knees

Focus
- ▶ Muscles of the shoulders and arms

Benefits
- ▶ Improves scapular mobility
- ▶ Activates and stabilizes the upper body
- ▶ Activates the core and promotes core awareness

1 Kneel with the arms bent, palms upward and in front of the body parallel to the floor. Place additional padding under the knees, if necessary. Knees can be together (more difficult for balance) or slightly separated at hip-width apart. The tailbone points downward along with the sit bones. Inhale and feel the shoulders press away from the ears, and feel the belly come in toward the spine to provide support for the lower back.

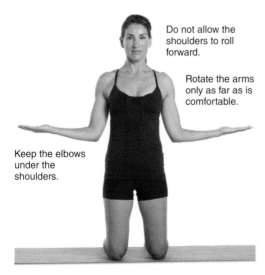

Do not allow the shoulders to roll forward.

Rotate the arms only as far as is comfortable.

Keep the elbows under the shoulders.

2 Exhale and rotate the forearms to the sides of the body.

3 Inhale and return the arms to the starting position. Repeat for 5 to 10 repetitions.

Oblique Crunch

Level
▶ Beginner

Contraindications
▶ Injuries to the knees or lower back

Focus
▶ Muscles of the trunk and spine

Benefits
▶ Strengthens the oblique abdominal muscles
▶ Creates awareness of the upper back
▶ Improves stability of the pelvis and hips

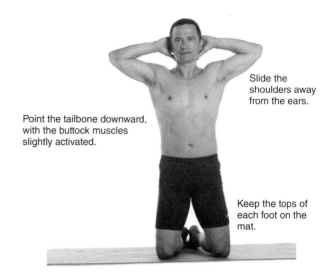

Slide the shoulders away from the ears.

Point the tailbone downward, with the buttock muscles slightly activated.

Keep the tops of each foot on the mat.

1 Kneel on the mat with the knees in line with the hip bones. (Place additional padding under the knees, if necessary.) Inhale and raise the arms over the head, and then exhale and bend the elbows, placing the hands behind the head. Inhale again as the body is prepared for upper body movement and abdominal engagement.

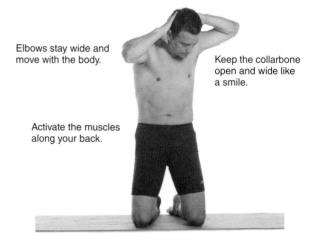

Elbows stay wide and move with the body.

Keep the collarbone open and wide like a smile.

Activate the muscles along your back.

2 Exhale and move the right rib cage to the left hip bone. Activate the muscles along each side of your back. Inhale to return to upright kneeling position, with the hands still behind the head.

3 Exhale and take the left rib cage toward the right hip bone. Inhale to return to the starting position. If you have trouble keeping your balance, tuck your toes under and press into the mat with your feet. Repeat for 6 to 10 repetitions on each side.

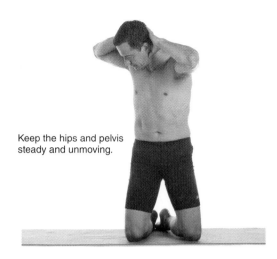

Keep the hips and pelvis steady and unmoving.

Cat-Cow

Level
▶ Beginner

Contraindications
▶ Injuries to the lower back, knees, or wrists

Focus
▶ Muscles of the spine and back

Benefits
▶ Increases spinal flexibility
▶ Stretches the lower, middle, and upper back
▶ Opens the front side of the body

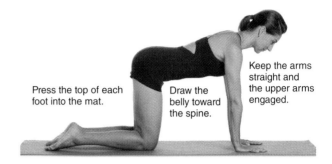

Press the top of each foot into the mat.

Draw the belly toward the spine.

Keep the arms straight and the upper arms engaged.

1 Kneel on all fours with the knees directly under the hips and the wrists under the shoulders. Inhale and lengthen the body from the top of the head to your tailbone, distributing the weight evenly to hands and knees, with fingers spread wide and pressing down.

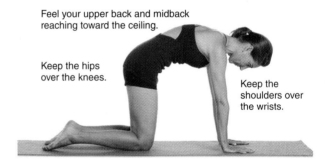

Feel your upper back and midback reaching toward the ceiling.

Keep the hips over the knees.

Keep the shoulders over the wrists.

2 Exhale and press into your hands. Round the spine, pulling the abdominals in deeper as if scooping inward. Tuck your pelvis under, and feel the pelvic floor engage and lift like an elevator toward the stomach and diaphragm. This is the cat position.

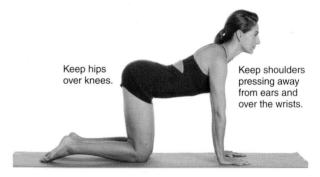

Keep hips over knees.

Keep shoulders pressing away from ears and over the wrists.

3 Inhale and tilt the tailbone toward the ceiling as the ribs and chest lower toward the floor. Lift the head, sternum, and eyes toward the ceiling. Repeat steps 2 and 3 for 5 to 10 breaths. Push back into Child's Pose (page 26), and rest the wrists and back for several breaths.

Tail Wag

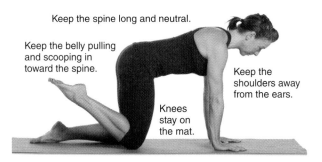

Keep the spine long and neutral.

Keep the belly pulling and scooping in toward the spine.

Keep the shoulders away from the ears.

Knees stay on the mat.

1 From the all-fours position and keeping both knees on the mat, lift your right shin with the toes pointed away from the body as you inhale.

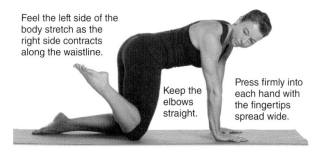

Feel the left side of the body stretch as the right side contracts along the waistline.

Keep the elbows straight.

Press firmly into each hand with the fingertips spread wide.

2 Exhale and swing the right foot to the right as you bend your body to the right and look to the right foot. Keep the right knee on the mat as you move the lower leg.

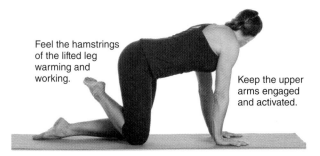

Feel the hamstrings of the lifted leg warming and working.

Keep the upper arms engaged and activated.

3 Inhale and swing the right foot to the left as you bend your body to the left and look toward the right foot. Continue this pattern for five to seven breaths, and then place the right foot down with an exhale. Inhale and repeat with the left foot for five to seven breaths, moving from left to right.

Level
▶ Beginner

Contraindications
▶ Injuries to the spine, knees, or wrists

Focus
▶ Muscles of the trunk and legs

Benefits
▶ Increases spinal lateral mobility
▶ Warms up the hamstrings and the sides of the body
▶ Activates the core

Sternum Drop

Level
▶ Beginner

Contraindications
▶ Injuries to the spine, knees, wrists, or shoulders

Focus
▶ Muscles of the shoulders and upper back

Benefits
▶ Promotes better posture
▶ Warms up and activates the shoulder girdle
▶ Mobilizes the shoulder blades along the rib cage

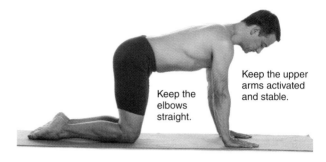

Keep the upper arms activated and stable.

Keep the elbows straight.

1 Kneel with the knees under the hips and the wrists under the shoulders. Create a long neutral spine and torso.

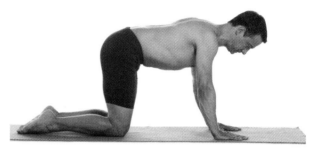

2 Inhale and allow the sternum and chest to lower toward the floor. The shoulder blades come toward one another across the upper back.

Keep the lower spine neutral and stable.

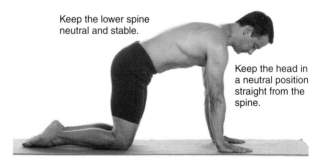

Keep the head in a neutral position straight from the spine.

3 Exhale and press into the hands as you lift your midback between the shoulder blades toward the ceiling. Imagine you have a suitcase handle between your shoulder blades, and someone just picked up the suitcase. The shoulder blades separate and spread wide across the upper back. Repeat for 6 to 10 repetitions.

Gentle Variation
If wrist injuries prevent you from doing this exercise, you can do the standing Shoulder Warming exercise (page 13) to get a similar feeling and warm up the shoulder girdle.

Kneeling Side Kick

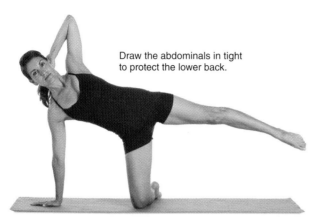

Draw the abdominals in tight to protect the lower back.

Keep the right arm straight and upper arm engaged.

Level
▶ Intermediate

Contraindications
▶ Injuries to the knees, wrists, or spine

Focus
▶ Muscles of the legs and hips

Benefits
▶ Stretches the hamstrings and hip flexors
▶ Strengthens and sculpts the outer thighs

1 Kneel on the mat with the right knee bent and the left leg stretched out from the hip. Place the left foot on the mat to the side of the left hip and the right hand on the mat in line with the right knee and under the right shoulder. Bend the left arm, and put the left hand behind the head. Inhale to prepare the abdominals. Feel them contract to protect the lower back. Exhale and lift the left leg to hip height straight out to the side.

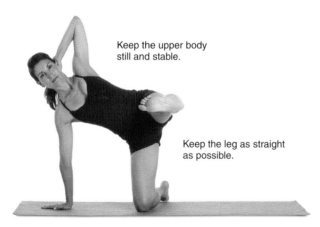

Keep the upper body still and stable.

Keep the leg as straight as possible.

2 Inhale with a double breath as you bring the left leg forward until you feel a stretch in the hamstrings. Keep the left leg straight and the foot flexed.

(continued)

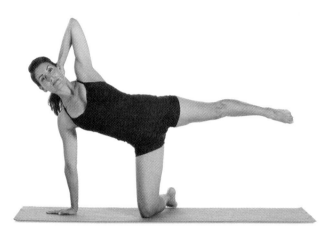

3 Exhale. Swing the left leg back at hip height with the toes pointed until you feel a stretch in the hip flexors. If your flexibility is limited, reduce your range of motion. Repeat for 10 repetitions with the left leg. Switch legs and repeat for 10 repetitions with the right leg.

Gentle Variation
Bend your knee slightly, if necessary.

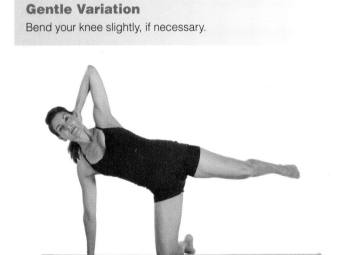

Chapter 4

Side-Lying Mat Exercises

There are three positions for lying mat exercises in Pilates: on the side, which is covered in this chapter; prone (lying on your abdomen), which is covered in chapter 5; and supine (lying on your back), which is covered in chapter 6. The side-lying exercises begin with a wonderful stretch for the shoulders and sides of the body and then continue with a very common side-lying exercise series that helps sculpt and shape the legs. This series can be done on one side completely and then repeated on the other side, or you can switch from one side to the other for each exercise. Even after gaining proficiency in each of the exercises, be sure to set up exactly like the first time so that you continue to feel the exercises and benefit from them.

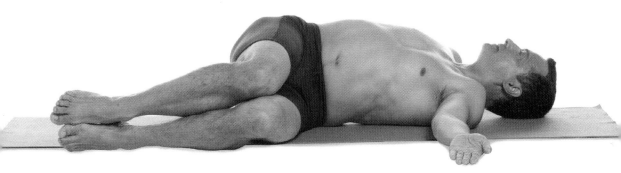

For the side-lying exercises, you may choose to use the standard position (figure 4.1) or one of the easier modifications (figures 4.2 and 4.3). When choosing which option to use for the side-lying exercises, comfort will be your first deciding factor. There can be a lot of pressure on the side of the hip and on the greater trochanter for some, and relieving this pressure is important in order to complete the exercises without strain and discomfort. Adding another mat under the body is always an option, but additional padding does not always help. Providing padding around the sensitive area with a hole for the greater trochanter to rest in will work for some but can prove difficult and cumbersome. Using the gentle modification shown in figure 4.3 will be easier and won't require purchasing more materials. It is also important to remember comfort of the neck area. Depending on the width of your shoulders, a prop might be necessary, as shown in figure 4.2, to bring the head in line with the neck and shoulders.

When you are lying on your side, remember to engage your core musculature and find a balance of the muscle engagement on either side of your trunk and spine. It should feel as if your torso is being propped up between two walls or panes of glass. This engagement of the core and trunk muscles will help you balance on your side and maintain the upper body in the correct position without tension. It is also important to maintain muscle engagement in the bottom leg to help with balance and to keep the torso and body in neutral alignment. This helps you take a mindful, full-body approach to these exercises and makes you work a bit harder.

For the standard side-lying position (figure 4.1), lie on your side and bring your legs down below your hips as if you were standing. Stack your feet, ankles, knees, and hips, and flex the feet as if you were standing on them. Now bring your legs just slightly in front of the body, creating a slight angle at the hips. Bring the arm closest to the floor above the head and under the ear. The palm can remain up or down, whichever is most comfortable.

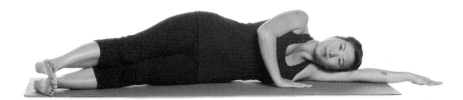

Figure 4.1   Standard side-lying position.

If your neck is tight or stiff, prop up your head on a pillow or block (figure 4.2). Use a small pillow or block because a large one will distort the line of the neck and head. The pillow or block should bring the head to a level position with the neck. This modification can be used when the arm is in front of the shoulders or when you are lying with that arm on the mat above the head.

If your lateral leg or greater trochanter is sensitive when you lie directly on the side of the leg, bend the bottom knee so that it is level with the hips (figure 4.3).

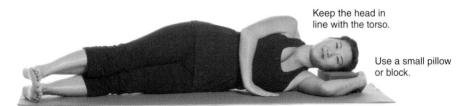

Keep the head in line with the torso.

Use a small pillow or block.

Figure 4.2 Gentle modification for side-lying position: head on a pillow or block.

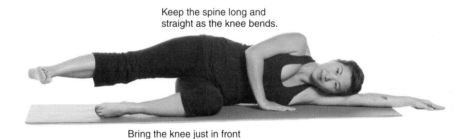

Keep the spine long and straight as the knee bends.

Bring the knee just in front of or just below the hip.

Figure 4.3 Gentle modification for side-lying position: bottom knee bent.

Pinwheel

Level
▶ Beginner

Contraindications
▶ Injuries to the shoulders or neck

Focus
▶ Muscles of the shoulders, upper back, and chest

Benefits
▶ Improves the mobility of the scapulae
▶ Helps coordinate the movement of the shoulder and scapula with upper body stability
▶ Stretches the chest and shoulders

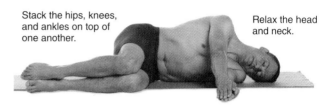

Stack the hips, knees, and ankles on top of one another.

Relax the head and neck.

1 Lie on your side with both knees bent in front of your hips. Align your back straight along the back edge of the mat. Take the arms out in front of your chest, stacking the hands one on top of the other. Allow the head to lie on the mat.

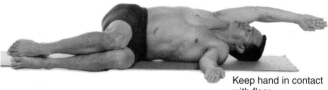

Pull abdominals in and up to support spine.

Keep hand in contact with floor.

2 Inhale and move your fingertips along the mat, tracing a semicircle over your head trying to keep the fingertips in touch with the mat. If the shoulders are tight, lift the arm off the mat where needed.

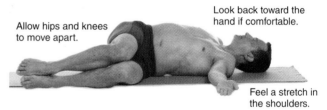

Look back toward the hand if comfortable.

Allow hips and knees to move apart.

Feel a stretch in the shoulders.

3 Continue the movement pattern with an exhale, making a semicircle above the head, bringing the fingertips as close to behind your back and shoulders as your flexibility allows. Keep the arm straight, and let the fingers lift off the mat if necessary. Move slowly and methodically to better stretch underneath the top arm and along the topside of your body.

4 Begin to inhale again, circling the arm and the fingertips back over the top of your head. Let the exhale complete the semicircle over the head, and restack the top hand over the bottom. Repeat for five to eight repetitions. Turn onto the other side and repeat.

Leg Lift

Feel the waist pull up from the ground and lengthen away from your ribs.

Flex the feet as if you were standing on them.

Bend the bottom elbow to cradle the head, if necessary.

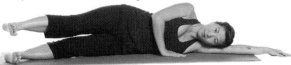

1 Lie on your side with your torso lined up straight along the back edge of the mat. Flex the hips so that the legs are slightly in front of your body. Stack the legs long and straight on top of one another, with the toes flexed toward the front. Your head lies over the bottom arm with the palm facing up or down. Bend the top elbow, and place the hand in front of the chest for support.

Feel the top leg reach away from the hip as it lifts off the bottom leg.

Flex at the hip and not at the waist when lifting the leg.

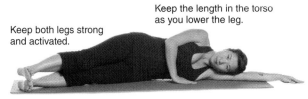

Keep the bottom leg contracted to help balance the body.

2 Inhale and lift the top leg up and off the bottom leg to hip height or just slightly above.

Keep the length in the torso as you lower the leg.

Keep both legs strong and activated.

3 Exhale and lower the leg back on top of the bottom leg. Repeat for 8 to 10 repetitions. You can go on to the next side-lying exercise on this side or switch sides and repeat the leg lift on the other side.

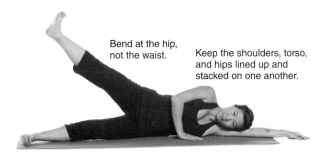

Bend at the hip, not the waist.

Keep the shoulders, torso, and hips lined up and stacked on one another.

Level
▶ Beginner

Contraindications
▶ Sensitivity in the outer hip area (greater trochanter)
▶ Injuries to the hips, neck, shoulders, elbows, or wrists

Focus
▶ Inner and outer thighs, external rotators

Benefits
▶ Improves control and stability in the hips, pelvis, and torso
▶ Strengthens the hip, butt, and lateral thigh muscles

Challenge
Turn out the top leg at the hip to allow the leg to lift as high as possible without shortening the waist.

Side-Lying Leg Circle

Level
▶ Beginner

Contraindications
▶ Sensitivity in the outer hip area (greater trochanter)
▶ Injuries to the hips, neck, shoulders, elbows, or wrists

Focus
▶ Inner and outer thighs, external rotators

Benefits
▶ Improves control and stability in the hips, pelvis, and torso
▶ Strengthens the hip, butt, and lateral thigh muscles

Flex the bottom foot as if you were standing on it.

Feel the waist pull up from the ground and lengthen away from your ribs.

Bend the bottom elbow to cradle the head, if necessary.

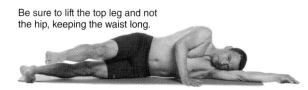

1 Lie on your side with your torso lined up straight along the back edge of the mat. Flex the hips so that the legs are slightly in front of your body. Stack the legs long and straight on top of one another, with the top toes pointed and the bottom toes flexed toward the front. Your head lies over the bottom arm with the palm facing up or down. Bend the top elbow, and place the hand in front of the body for support.

Be sure to lift the top leg and not the hip, keeping the waist long.

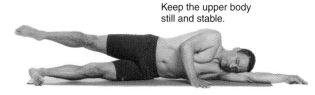

2 Inhale and circle the top leg forward and upward. Keep circles small—about the size of a dinner plate— to maintain stability in the torso.

Keep the upper body still and stable.

3 Exhale and continue to circle the top leg to the back and then down over the bottom leg. Circle in this frontal direction for 8 to 10 times, and then do 8 to 10 repetitions starting the circle to the back. You can go on to the next side-lying exercise on this side or switch sides and repeat the leg circle on the other side, with circles in each direction.

Front Kick

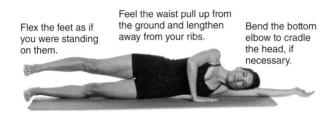

Flex the feet as if you were standing on them.

Feel the waist pull up from the ground and lengthen away from your ribs.

Bend the bottom elbow to cradle the head, if necessary.

1 Lie on your side with your torso lined up straight along the back edge of the mat. Flex the hips so that the legs are slightly in front of your body. Stack the legs long and straight on top of one another, with the toes flexed toward the front. Your head lies over the bottom arm with the palm facing up or down. Bend the top elbow, and place the hand in front of the body for support.

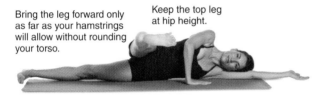

Bring the leg forward only as far as your hamstrings will allow without rounding your torso.

Keep the top leg at hip height.

2 Using a sniffing breath, inhale two times as you kick the top leg forward with a double pulse. Keep the top foot flexed to intensify the stretch.

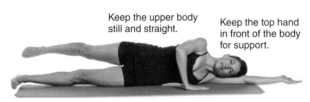

Keep the upper body still and straight.

Keep the top hand in front of the body for support.

Use the abdominals to stabilize the torso.

3 Exhale and bring the top leg back, with the toes pointed, behind the hip as far as the hip flexors will allow without rounding or changing the torso position. Repeat the kicks for 8 to 10 repetitions. You can go on to the next side-lying exercise on this side or switch sides and repeat the front kick on the other side.

Level

▶ Intermediate

Contraindications

▶ Sensitivity in the outer hip area (greater trochanter)

▶ Injuries to the hips, neck, shoulders, elbows, or wrists

Focus

▶ Inner and outer thighs, external rotators, hamstrings, and hip flexors

Benefits

▶ Improves control and stability in the hips, pelvis, and torso

▶ Strengthens the hip, butt, and lateral thigh muscles

▶ Stretches the hamstrings and hip flexors

Leg Tap

Level

► Intermediate

Contraindications

► Sensitivity in the outer hip area (greater trochanter)
► Injuries to the hips, neck, shoulders, elbows, or wrists

Focus

► Inner and outer thighs, external rotators, hamstrings, hip flexors, and buttocks

Benefits

► Improves control and stability in the hips, pelvis, and torso
► Strengthens the hip, butt, and lateral thigh muscles

Flex the bottom foot as if you were standing on it.

Feel the waist pull up from the ground and lengthen away from your ribs.

Bend the bottom elbow to cradle the head, if necessary.

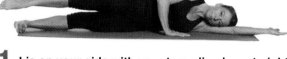

1 Lie on your side with your torso lined up straight along the back edge of the mat. Flex the hips so that the legs are slightly in front of your body. Stack the legs long and straight on top of one another, with the top toes pointed and the bottom toes flexed toward the front. Your head lies over the bottom arm with the palm facing up or down. Bend the top elbow, and place the hand in front of the body for support.

Keep the rib cage pulling away from the mat.

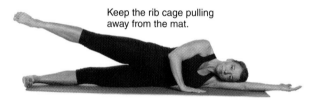

2 Inhale to lift the top leg up above the hips. Lift the leg only as high as you can without collapsing the rib cage toward the mat.

Keep the upper body steady and still.

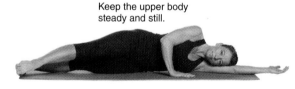

3 Bring the foot down a few inches or centimeters in front of the bottom foot. Use a strong double exhale and double tap to bring the focus to the inner thighs.

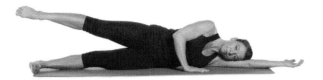

4 Inhale to lift the top leg up above the hips. Lift the leg only as high as you can without collapsing the rib cage toward the mat.

Focus on the inner thighs as you lower the top leg.

Keep the upper body still and the breath strong and focused.

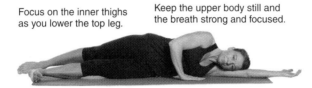

5 Use a strong double exhale as you bring the foot down a few inches or centimeters behind the bottom foot with a double tap. Repeat for 5 to 10 repetitions. You can go on to the last side-lying exercise on this side or switch to the other side and repeat the leg tap on the other side.

Side-Lying Bicycle

Level

▶ Intermediate

Contraindications

▶ Sensitivity in the outer hip area (greater trochanter)
▶ Injuries to the hips, neck, shoulders, elbows, or wrists

Focus

▶ Inner and outer thighs, external rotators, hamstrings, hip flexors, and buttocks

Benefits

▶ Improves control and stability in the hips, pelvis, and torso
▶ Strengthens the hip, butt, and lateral thigh muscles
▶ Stretches the hip flexors and hamstrings

Flex the bottom foot as if you were standing on it.

Feel the waist pull up from the ground and lengthen away from your ribs.

Bend the bottom elbow to cradle the head, if necessary.

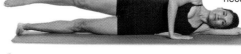

1 Lie on your side with your torso lined up straight along the back edge of the mat. Flex the hips so that the legs are slightly in front of your body. Stack the legs long and straight on top of one another, with the top toes pointed and the bottom toes flexed toward the front. Your head lies over the bottom arm with the palm facing up or down. Bend the top elbow, and place the hand in front of the body for support.

Keep the top leg at hip height only.

Keep the torso straight as the knee lifts toward the hips.

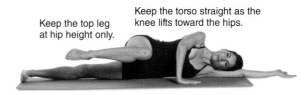

2 Inhale and bend the top leg, bringing the knee in front of the hips and parallel to the floor. If your hamstrings are tight, bend the knee to just below the hip only.

Keep the torso long and straight as the leg straightens to the front.

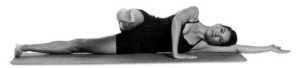

3 Continue to inhale as you extend and straighten the top leg in front of the hips. If your hamstrings are tight, keep the knee slightly bent.

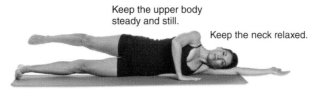

Keep the upper body
steady and still.

Keep the neck relaxed.

4 Exhale and swing the leg back over the bottom leg and behind the hips, keeping the leg as straight as possible.

Keep the upper body from
rocking forward or backward.

Be sure to do the same
number of repetitions to the
front as you do to the back.

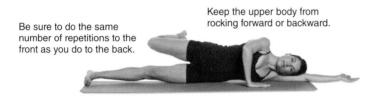

5 Continue to exhale as the top leg bends behind the hips. Repeat for five to eight repetitions in a forward direction and then reverse the bicycle, starting the pattern to the back. If you have been switching sides with each side-lying exercise, switch sides and repeat the bicycle on the other side. If you have been working through all the side-lying exercises on the same side, switch to the other side now and complete the full cycle of side-lying leg exercises, starting with the Leg Lift (page 39).

Chapter 5

Prone Mat Exercises

Prone mat exercises are great for strengthening the entire back musculature. A strong back is important for correct posture and to help alleviate lower back pain. Pay particular attention to the setup and modifications if you have a sensitive lower back or previous injuries or conditions. Also remember to engage the lower abdominals throughout each exercise to ensure that the lower back is supported and safe. When finished with any or all of the prone exercises, perform the Child's Pose exercise from chapter 3 (page 26) to stretch and rest the lower spine.

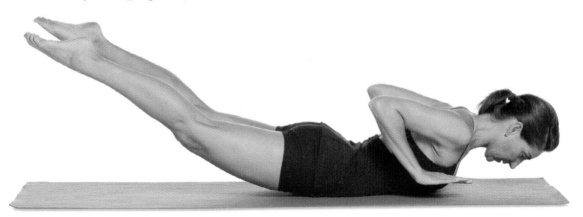

Oppositional Stretch

Level
▶ Beginner

Contraindications
▶ Pain in or injuries to the lower back, shoulders, or legs

Focus
▶ Hamstrings and muscles of the back, shoulders, and core

Benefits
▶ Strengthens the hamstrings, back extensors, and buttocks
▶ Lengthens the torso
▶ Mobilizes the shoulders and arms
▶ Activates the core muscles

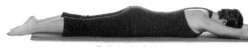

Draw the shoulder blades away from the ears and down the back.

Feel long, like a snake on the mat.

Pull the belly button toward the spine.

1 Lie on your abdomen with the arms stretched above the head, palms down, and legs stretched out with the tops of the feet on the mat. Legs are sit-bone-distance apart. Inhale to prepare.

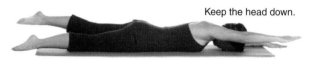

Keep the head down.

2 Exhale. Lift one arm and the opposite leg slightly off the mat. Think of length and not height. Lift the arm and leg only slightly. Feel as if you were being pulled in opposite directions.

Keep the length in the body as the arm and leg lower.

Pull the belly upward.

3 Inhale as you lower the arm and leg to the mat.

Feel yourself lengthening and stretching further with each repetition.

Press the shoulders away from the ears and down the back.

Keep your head on the mat.

4 Exhale and lift the other arm and opposite leg. Inhale as you return the arm and leg to the mat. Repeat for four to six sets, alternating sides.

Thigh Stretch

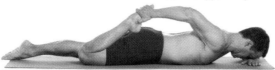

Relax the upper body.

Pull the belly button
toward the spine.

1 Lie on your abdomen with one arm bent and the hand underneath your forehead. With the other hand, grab the top of the foot on the same side as you bend the knee to bring the foot toward the buttocks. Legs are sit-bone-distance apart. Inhale to prepare.

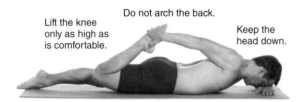

Do not arch the back.

Lift the knee
only as high as
is comfortable.

Keep the
head down.

2 Exhale as you press the foot into the hand, lifting the knee slightly off the mat. You will feel the stretch in the front of the bent leg. Hold the stretch for 30 to 45 seconds. Switch sides and repeat.

Level
▶ Beginner

Contraindications
▶ Pain in or injuries to the lower back, arms, legs, or knees

Focus
▶ Thighs, back, shoulders, and hips

Benefits
▶ Stretches the quadriceps
▶ Stretches the muscles that support the knees
▶ Strengthens the back muscles
▶ Activates the core muscles

Single-Leg Kick

Level
▶ Beginner

Contraindications
▶ Pain in or injuries to the lower back, shoulders, elbows, or knees

Focus
▶ Hamstrings, upper back, shoulders, and abdominals

Benefits
▶ Strengthens the hamstrings
▶ Strengthens the upper back
▶ Stretches and strengthens the abdominals
▶ Stretches the quadriceps
▶ Improves shoulder stability

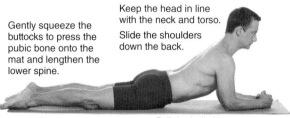

Keep the head in line with the neck and torso.

Gently squeeze the buttocks to press the pubic bone onto the mat and lengthen the lower spine.

Slide the shoulders down the back.

Pull the belly button in toward the spine.

1 Lie on your abdomen with the head and torso lifted off the mat. Place your forearms on the mat directly underneath your shoulders, and press into the elbows to lift up through your chest.

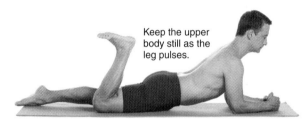

Keep the upper body still as the leg pulses.

2 Inhale and bend one knee, pulsing the heel toward the buttocks two times with the foot flexed. Exhale to straighten the leg to start position.

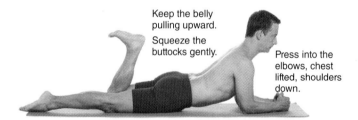

Keep the belly pulling upward.
Squeeze the buttocks gently.

Press into the elbows, chest lifted, shoulders down.

3 Inhale and bend the other knee, pulsing the heel toward the buttocks two times with the foot flexed. Exhale to straighten the leg to the start position. Repeat, alternating legs each time, for 8 to 10 sets.

Gentle Modification
If the shoulders are not strong or there is an injury, fold the hands over each other and place them in front of the shoulders. Lay the forehead on the back of the hands.

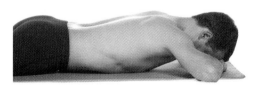

Belly keeps pulling away from the mat even if it is touching.

Swimming

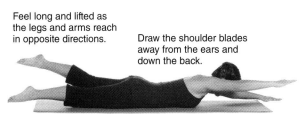

Feel long and lifted as the legs and arms reach in opposite directions.

Draw the shoulder blades away from the ears and down the back.

Pull the belly button toward the spine.

1 **Lie on your abdomen with the arms stretched above the head, palms turned down, and slightly lifted off the mat. One arm is just above shoulder height and the other is just below. Lift the legs, one just above hip height and one slightly below. Keep the legs separated about hip-distance apart. Inhale deeply to prepare.**

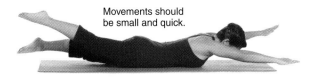

Movements should be small and quick.

2 **Exhale for five counts as you flutter kick the legs and arms in opposition in tiny movements.**

3 **Inhale for five counts, continuing to flutter kick the arms and legs. Keep the spine long. Pull the abdominals up and in. Repeat for four to six breaths.**

Gentle Variation

As an option, make the flutter kicks and breath slow and methodical.

Level
► Beginner to intermediate

Contraindications
► Pain in or injuries to the lower back, shoulders, or legs

Focus
► Hamstrings and muscles of the back, shoulders, and core

Benefits
► Strengthens the hamstrings, back extensors, and buttocks
► Lengthens the torso
► Mobilizes the shoulders and arms
► Activates the core muscles
► Teaches coordination and balance

Double-Leg Kick

Level
▶ Intermediate

Contraindications
▶ Pain in or injuries to the lower back, shoulders, elbows, or knees

Focus
▶ Hamstrings, upper back, shoulders

Benefits
▶ Strengthens the hamstrings
▶ Strengthens the upper back
▶ Stretches the chest
▶ Stretches the quadriceps
▶ Improves shoulder stability, mobility, and flexibility

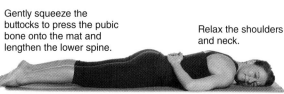

Gently squeeze the buttocks to press the pubic bone onto the mat and lengthen the lower spine.

Relax the shoulders and neck.

Pull the belly button toward the spine.

1 Lie on your abdomen with your arms bent and hands placed behind your back. Turn your head to one side, pressing your ear to the mat. Your inner thighs are sit-bone-distance apart. Contract the muscles in both legs, and draw the belly in away from the mat.

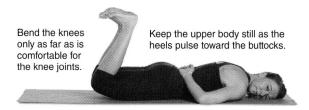

Bend the knees only as far as is comfortable for the knee joints.

Keep the upper body still as the heels pulse toward the buttocks.

2 With a double inhale, bend both knees, kicking the heels toward the buttocks with a double breath. Keep your head turned to one side when inhaling.

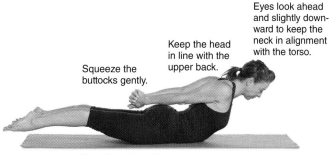

Eyes look ahead and slightly downward to keep the neck in alignment with the torso.

Keep the head in line with the upper back.

Squeeze the buttocks gently.

Keep the belly pulling upward.

3 Exhale. Straighten and lift both legs off the ground as you straighten both arms, hands still clasped behind the back, and lift the upper body.

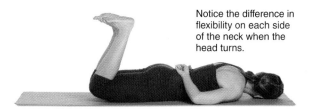

Notice the difference in flexibility on each side of the neck when the head turns.

4 Inhale and bend both knees again as you lower the upper body and turn your head in the opposite direction. Bend your arms, and bring your hands to the lower back as your head lowers and knees bend. Repeat for four to six sets.

Gentle Modification

If your shoulders and wrists are tight, keep your arms alongside the body when lifting and lowering the upper body.

Activate and contract the upper arms as the body lifts on the exhale.

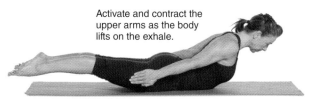

Arms lie on the mat beside the body as you inhale and bend the knees.

Swan

Level
▶ Intermediate

Contraindications
▶ Pain in or injuries to the lower back, shoulders, elbows, or wrists

Focus
▶ Hamstrings, upper back, shoulders

Benefits
▶ Strengthens the hamstrings, back extensors, and buttocks
▶ Stretches the abdominals
▶ Improves shoulder stability
▶ Increases range of motion in back extension

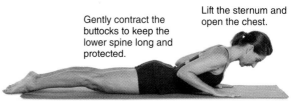

Draw the shoulder blades away from the ears and down the back.

Pull the belly button in toward the spine.

1 Lie on your abdomen, with the elbows bent and hands on the mat in front of and outside the tops of the shoulders. The forehead is on the mat. Inner thighs are sit-bone-distance apart, with both legs contracted and the belly drawn in away from the mat. Gently squeeze the buttocks to press the pubic bone onto the mat and lengthen the lower spine.

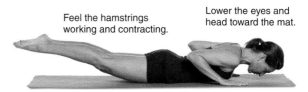

Gently contract the buttocks to keep the lower spine long and protected.

Lift the sternum and open the chest.

Straighten arms only as far as is comfortable for the lower spine.

2 Inhale and press into the hands as you lift your upper body.

Feel the hamstrings working and contracting.

Lower the eyes and head toward the mat.

Keep the belly pulling upward.

3 Exhale as you lower the upper body to the mat, lifting the legs toward the ceiling. Repeat for four to six times. If your back is not tired, continue to the challenge move.

Challenge
After step 3, inhale and press into the hands as you lift your upper body and lower the legs to the floor (same as step 2). Exhale and lift your hands off the floor, lowering the upper body and lifting the legs off the floor. Another option (not shown) is to reach forward with the arms, which are slightly lifted from the floor, as you rock forward. Repeat for four to six repetitions.

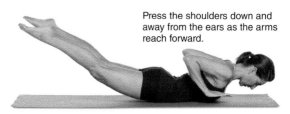

Press the shoulders down and away from the ears as the arms reach forward.

Pull the belly toward the spine throughout the exercise.

Push-Up

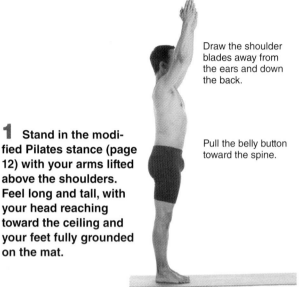

Draw the shoulder blades away from the ears and down the back.

1 Stand in the modi- fied Pilates stance (page 12) with your arms lifted above the shoulders. Feel long and tall, with your head reaching toward the ceiling and your feet fully grounded on the mat.

Pull the belly button toward the spine.

Level
▶ Intermediate to advanced

Contraindications
▶ Pain in or injuries to the lower back, shoulders, elbows, or wrists

Focus
▶ Muscles of the arms, abdominals, legs, and hips

Benefits
▶ Strengthens the entire body

2 Inhale and bring the chin toward the chest. Roll down the spine one vertebra at a time, reaching the arms toward the mat. Bend the knees as needed as the hands reach for the mat.

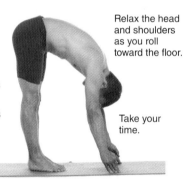

Relax the head and shoulders as you roll toward the floor.

Take your time.

Pull the shoulder blades away from the ears and down the back.

Keep the body elongated.

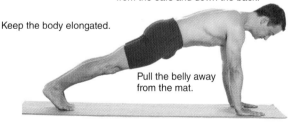

Pull the belly away from the mat.

3 Exhale as you walk the hands out in front of the body until you are in plank position, with each wrist underneath each shoulder. As a modification, you can hold this position for several breaths and then continue from step 6 to the end.

(continued)

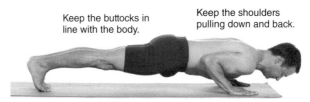

Keep the buttocks in line with the body.

Keep the shoulders pulling down and back.

Feel the elbows scrape the rib cage.

4 Inhale and bend your elbows downward and backward as you lower your body toward the mat.

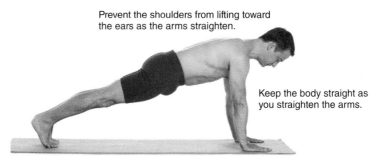

Prevent the shoulders from lifting toward the ears as the arms straighten.

Keep the body straight as you straighten the arms.

5 Exhale and straighten the arms, pressing the body away from the mat. Repeat steps 4 and 5 for 4 to 10 repetitions.

6 Inhale and walk the hands back toward the feet. Exhale as you restack the spine and stand up tall, arms by your sides.

Modification
Keep the knees bent and on the mat as you bend and straighten the arms in the push-up position.

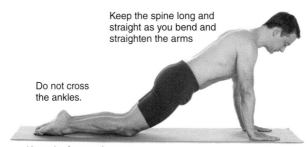

Keep the spine long and straight as you bend and straighten the arms

Do not cross the ankles.

Keep the feet on the mat.

Chapter 6

Supine Mat Exercises

Most Pilates exercises fall into this category. Ideally supine mat exercises feature a balance of strength and flexibility in the abdominals and lower back. Finding a balance between the strength and flexibility of the torso is critical for creating ease of movement and good posture overall as well as for limiting the compression on the spine itself during exercise and while at rest. Building the strength of your abdominals and your back means you are building a strong core, and this is the ultimate goal of Pilates.

Supine mat exercises use one of three basic starting positions for the pelvis and lower spine: the neutral pelvis, the imprinted spine, and the supported neutral spine. Some may find it more comfortable to support the head as well. A small pillow or bath towel under the head will help keep the neck in proper position.

In the neutral pelvis position (figure 6.1), the lower spine forms its own natural curve. This position will vary from person to person depending on musculature, body size, and the amount of flesh and tissue in the midsection. For some, when in this position the lower spine is lifted slightly off the mat in its natural curvature. For others, when in this position the lower back is touching the floor. Ideally, the top of the pelvis (the anterior superior iliac spine, or ASIS) and the pubic bone form a level triangle with the mat. Rock gently back and forth between anterior and posterior pelvis positioning to find a comfortable and natural position. This position should not stress the lower spine or anywhere else. This is the position to use if you have no special spinal conditions or pain.

Note: In figures 6.1 through 6.3, the arms are lifted over the head to show a clear view of the spine and spinal placement. When practicing these positions, keep your arms down by your sides with the palms turned down.

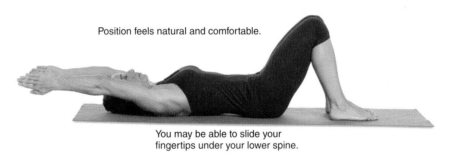

Position feels natural and comfortable.

You may be able to slide your
fingertips under your lower spine.

Figure 6.1 Neutral pelvis position. The natural curve of the lower spine is shown. The ASIS and pubic bone form a level triangle with the mat.

In the imprinted spine position (figure 6.2), the lower spine flexes forward slightly, lengthening the lumbar spine to protect the back. In most cases, though not all, the lower spine will actually touch the mat. Use the imprinted spine position when you feel a weakness in the core or if you experience pain in the lower spine. Some conditions do not tolerate an imprinted spine, so please consult with your doctor if you are unsure.

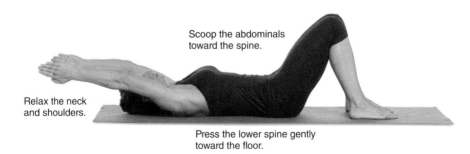

Scoop the abdominals
toward the spine.

Relax the neck
and shoulders.

Press the lower spine gently
toward the floor.

Figure 6.2 Imprinted spine position. The lower spine flexes forward slightly.

The supported neutral position (figure 6.3) is ideal for someone with an excessive curve in the lumbar (lower) spine because it supports the spine during movement and does not allow the lower back to move through an excessive range of motion, which could cause discomfort. For those with an excessive curve in the lower spine, placing the lower spine on the mat may be impossible, uncomfortable, and dangerous. Place a small rolled-up towel (or my favorite, a roll of shelf lining from a kitchen supply center) under the small of the back. Use enough material to prop up the lower spine but not so much that it obstructs proper movement. This will keep you from stressing the upper body or buttocks as you try to place the lower spine on the mat.

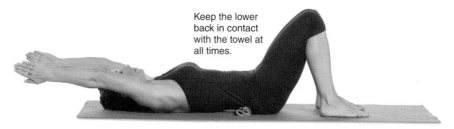

Keep the lower back in contact with the towel at all times.

Figure 6.3 Supported neutral position. A small rolled-up towel under the small of the back prevents excessive stress on the upper body or buttocks.

Supine Leg Circle

Level
▶ Beginner

Contraindications
▶ Pain in, injuries to, or chronic conditions of the lower back or hips

Focus
▶ Abdominals and muscles of the legs and scapulae

Benefits
▶ Increases flexibility of the hips and legs
▶ Warms up the hip joint and pelvis
▶ Builds awareness of the scapular musculature and stability
▶ Strengthens the abdominals

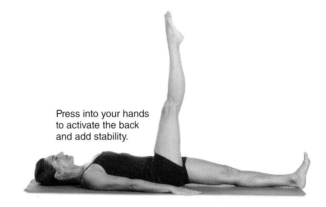

Press into your hands to activate the back and add stability.

1 Lie on your back with your arms by your sides, palms down, and one leg extended over the hip. The toes of the lifted leg are pointed toward the ceiling. The foot of the leg on the mat is flexed.

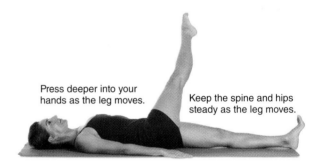

Press deeper into your hands as the leg moves.

Keep the spine and hips steady as the leg moves.

2 Inhale as you move the lifted leg partially across the grounded leg.

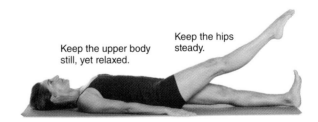

Keep the upper body still, yet relaxed.

Keep the hips steady.

3 Continue to inhale as the leg circles down at an angle. This is the first half of a circular movement pattern.

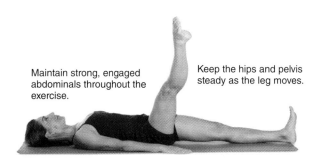

Maintain strong, engaged abdominals throughout the exercise.

Keep the hips and pelvis steady as the leg moves.

4 **Exhale as you bring the lifted leg outside the body and then up and around to the start position above the hip. This is the finish position of the circling pattern. Repeat for 5 to 10 times in this direction. Reverse the direction of the circle, following the same pattern for 5 to 10 times. Then switch legs and repeat on the other side.**

Gentle Modification

Bend the lifted leg either at a slight angle or a full 90 degrees as shown.

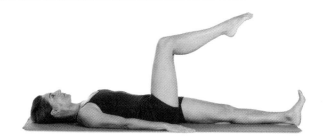

Pelvic Peel

Level
▶ Beginner

Contraindications
▶ Pain in, injuries to, or chronic conditions of the trunk or shoulders

Focus
▶ Muscles of the back, legs, and arms

Benefits
▶ Strengthens the back extensor muscles
▶ Strengthens the leg muscles, especially the hamstrings
▶ Increases core stability and strength
▶ Mobilizes the spine and pelvis
▶ Activates the core

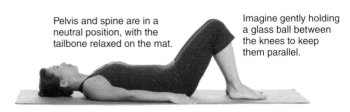

Pelvis and spine are in a neutral position, with the tailbone relaxed on the mat.

Imagine gently holding a glass ball between the knees to keep them parallel.

1 Lie on your back with the knees bent and heels in line with your sit bones. Hands are palms down on the mat by your sides. Inhale. You will remain in this neutral position with the spine and pelvis.

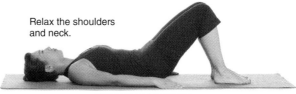

Relax the shoulders and neck.

Scoop the abdominals inward toward the mat.

2 Exhale as you tuck the pelvis under and lightly press the spine to the mat.

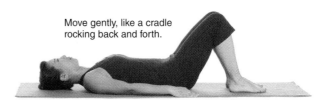

Move gently, like a cradle rocking back and forth.

3 Inhale as you return to the start position. Repeat from step 2 for four to six repetitions. Note: If you are using a towel or other prop to support your head, remove it before moving into step 4.

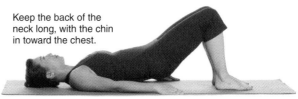

Keep the back of the neck long, with the chin in toward the chest.

As the hips press up, keep the pelvis neutral and stable.

4 After the last repetition of step 3, curl the tailbone under and lift the hips sequentially one vertebra at a time as you exhale.

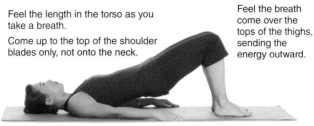

Feel the length in the torso as you take a breath.

Come up to the top of the shoulder blades only, not onto the neck.

Feel the breath come over the tops of the thighs, sending the energy outward.

Keep the pelvis in line with the shoulders and the knees.

5 Inhale as you hold the hips at the top of the bridge.

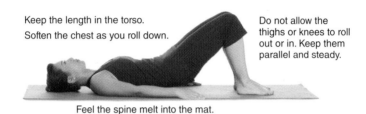

Keep the length in the torso.

Soften the chest as you roll down.

Do not allow the thighs or knees to roll out or in. Keep them parallel and steady.

Feel the spine melt into the mat.

6 Exhale as you slowly roll down the spine.

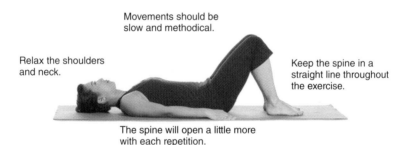

Movements should be slow and methodical.

Relax the shoulders and neck.

Keep the spine in a straight line throughout the exercise.

The spine will open a little more with each repetition.

7 Inhale and stay in this neutral position. Repeat from step 4 for four to six repetitions.

Hundred

Level
▶ Beginner to intermediate

Contraindications
▶ Pain in, injuries to, or chronic conditions of the trunk

Focus
▶ Abdominals and muscles of the arms and legs

Benefits
▶ Warms up the body
▶ Teaches correct breathing with abdominal engagement
▶ Increases abdominal strength
▶ Increases upper back flexibility
▶ Teaches correct position for the head in all upper body lifts (abdominal exercises)

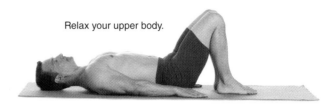

Relax your upper body.

1 Lie on your back with the knees bent and feet on the floor, heels in line with the sit bones. Use the neutral pelvis, imprinted spine, or supported natural spine position, depending on your needs. Arms are by your sides, palms turned down. This is the common starting position for most abdominal-based exercises in this book.

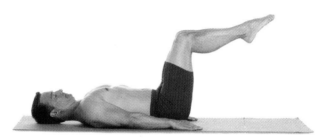

2 Inhale and lift one knee above the hip. Exhale and lift the other knee above the hip. (This is also known as tabletop position.) Inhale and lower the chin toward (but not onto) the chest to lengthen the neck.

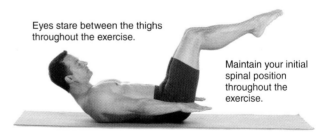

Eyes stare between the thighs throughout the exercise.

Maintain your initial spinal position throughout the exercise.

3 Exhale and lift the upper body by flexing the upper spine forward. Allow the arms to float off the mat. You may choose to stay here to do the exercise or try the challenge position. Inhale and pulse the arms for five counts (approximately 5 seconds) as the upper body stays still. Exhale and pulse the arms for five counts (approximately 5 seconds). Repeat for 10 repetitions or breaths.

Challenge

To make the hundred more challenging, extend the legs from tabletop position to a 45-degree angle from the body.

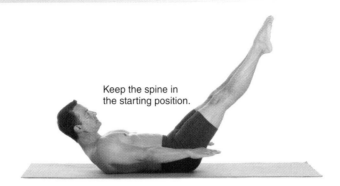

Keep the spine in the starting position.

Gentle Modification

Straighten the legs above the hips instead of holding them at a 45-degree angle if your lower back lifts off the mat. Bend your knees slightly if your hamstrings are tight.

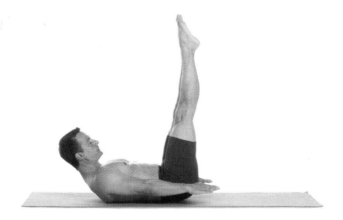

Roll-Up

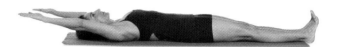

Level
▶ Beginner to intermediate

Contraindications
▶ Pain in, injuries to, or chronic conditions of the neck or trunk

Focus
▶ Abdominals and muscles of the back and scapulae

Benefits
▶ Strengthens the abdominals
▶ Increases lower back flexibility
▶ Teaches spinal articulation

1 Lie down on the mat with the arms extended above the head. The arms might touch the floor or might not, depending on the flexibility of the shoulders or any tightness in the upper back. If the lower back is tight, use the supported neutral starting position, as this will aid you in rolling through the tightness in the lower spine. Inner thighs are together, and feet can be pointed or flexed depending on comfort.

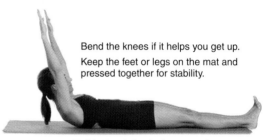

Bend the knees if it helps you get up.
Keep the feet or legs on the mat and pressed together for stability.

Pull in the abdominals to stretch and support the lower spine.

2 Inhale and lift the arms to the ceiling. Bring the chin toward the chest as you roll the head and then the spine off the mat, rising one vertebra at a time.

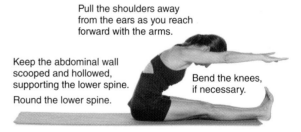

Pull the shoulders away from the ears as you reach forward with the arms.

Keep the abdominal wall scooped and hollowed, supporting the lower spine.
Round the lower spine.

Bend the knees, if necessary.

3 Exhale as you continue to roll up and forward until the arms are parallel with the floor and over the legs.

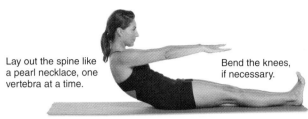

Lay out the spine like a pearl necklace, one vertebra at a time.

Bend the knees, if necessary.

Focus on stretching the lower spine to reach the mat.

4 Inhale as you begin to roll back, keeping the arms in front of the chest as you lower your upper body.

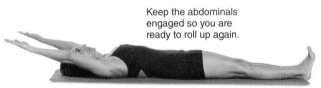

Keep the abdominals engaged so you are ready to roll up again.

Press the lower back part of the rib cage down into the mat.

5 Exhale and continue to roll down until the arms are over the head and the head is on the mat. Repeat for five to eight times.

Single-Leg Stretch

Level
▶ Beginner to intermediate

Contraindications
▶ Pain in, injuries to, or chronic conditions of the trunk or shoulders

Focus
▶ Abdominals and muscles of the back

Benefits
▶ Strengthens the abdominals
▶ Increases upper back flexibility
▶ Teaches core control
▶ Teaches breath and movement coordination

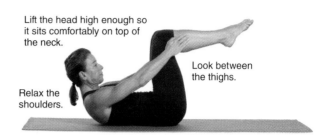

Lift the head high enough so it sits comfortably on top of the neck.

Relax the shoulders.

Look between the thighs.

1 Lie on your back with your knees above the hips in tabletop position and the upper body lifted, arms reaching out by the knees. Inhale to prepare.

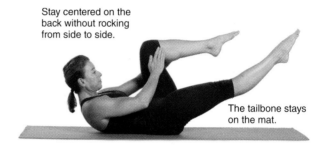

Stay centered on the back without rocking from side to side.

The tailbone stays on the mat.

2 Exhale as you extend one leg to a 45-degree angle from the mat and draw the other knee in toward the chest. The fingertips of the hand on the same side as the bent knee reach toward that ankle as the other hand guides the knee toward the chest. Keep your tailbone on the mat. Stop drawing in the knee if your tailbone lifts off the mat.

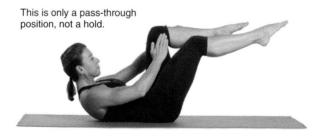

This is only a pass-through position, not a hold.

3 Inhale as you begin to bring the straight leg back toward tabletop position and the tabletop leg to an extended position, keeping the head in place above the neck.

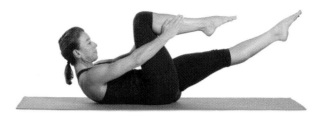

4 Exhale as you extend the other leg to a 45-degree angle from the mat, drawing the other knee toward the chest. The fingertips of the hand on the same side as the bent knee reach toward that ankle as the other hand guides the knee toward the chest. Repeat, alternating legs, for 5 to 10 sets.

Gentle Modification

If the neck gets sore or is unable to hold up the head, keep the head down throughout the exercise. Or prop up your head with a pillow or a folded towel to support the neck. If you use this option, you may keep the hands by your sides to support the back or reach for the legs as in the standard version.

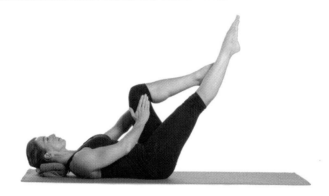

Double-Leg Stretch

Level

▷ Beginner to intermediate

Contraindications

▷ Pain in, injuries to, or chronic conditions of the trunk or shoulders

Focus

▷ Abdominals and muscles of the legs, arms, and back

Benefits

▷ Strengthens the abdominals
▷ Increases upper back flexibility
▷ Teaches core control
▷ Teaches breath and movement coordination

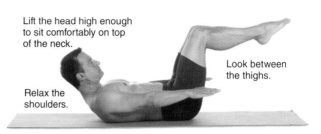

Lift the head high enough to sit comfortably on top of the neck.

Relax the shoulders.

Look between the thighs.

1 **Lie on your back with your knees above the hips in tabletop position and the upper body lifted and arms reaching out by the knees.**

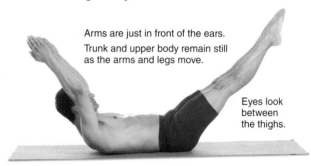

Arms are just in front of the ears. Trunk and upper body remain still as the arms and legs move.

Eyes look between the thighs.

Belly presses in toward the spine.

2 **Inhale as you extend both legs out at a 45-degree angle and raise your arms up by the ears. Keep your arms just in front of your ears to keep the head in place and prevent neck strain.**

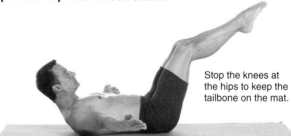

Stop the knees at the hips to keep the tailbone on the mat.

3 **Exhale as you draw the knees back to tabletop position above the hips and circle the arms around and back to the start position. Repeat for 5 to 10 times.**

Gentle Modification

Keep the knees bent, and tap the toes gently on the mat as the arms circle around. If necessary, make the arm circles smaller.

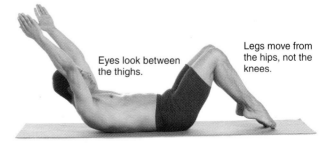

Eyes look between the thighs.

Legs move from the hips, not the knees.

Single Straight-Leg Stretch

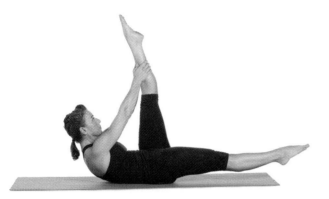

Level
- ▶ Intermediate

Contraindications
- ▶ Pain in, injuries to, or chronic conditions of the trunk or shoulders

Focus
- ▶ Abdominals and muscles of the legs, arms, and back

Benefits
- ▶ Strengthens the abdominals
- ▶ Increases upper back and hamstring flexibility
- ▶ Teaches core control
- ▶ Teaches breath and movement coordination

1 Lie on your back with one leg reaching toward the ceiling and the other leg stretched from the hip above the mat. Lift your head, and reach with both arms toward the lifted leg, holding onto the calf from behind. If your flexibility is limited, you may take hold of the leg above the knee.

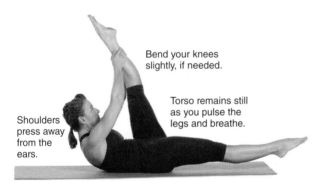

Bend your knees slightly, if needed.

Torso remains still as you pulse the legs and breathe.

Shoulders press away from the ears.

2 Pull the lifted leg toward you as the leg parallel to the mat pulses away from you and you inhale quickly two times.

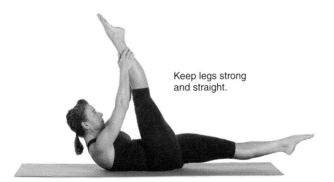

Keep legs strong and straight.

3 Exhale as you switch legs. Repeat the sequence with the new leg positions. Repeat, alternating legs, for 5 to 10 sets.

Double Straight-Leg Stretch

Level
▶ Intermediate

Contraindications
▶ Pain in, injuries to, or chronic conditions of the neck, torso, or shoulders

Focus
▶ Abdominals and muscles of the legs, arms, and back

Benefits
▶ Strengthens the abdominals
▶ Increases upper back flexibility
▶ Teaches core control
▶ Teaches breath and movement coordination

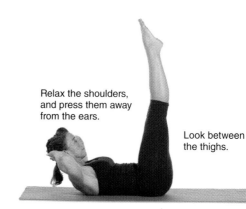

Relax the shoulders, and press them away from the ears.

Look between the thighs.

1 Lie on your back with your legs straight above the hips and the upper body lifted, head supported by the hands and the elbows wide beside the ears.

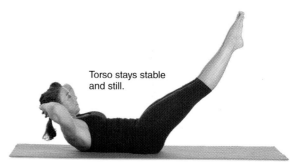

Torso stays stable and still.

Keep the spine in the start position.

2 Inhale as you lower both legs to a 45-degree angle above the floor.

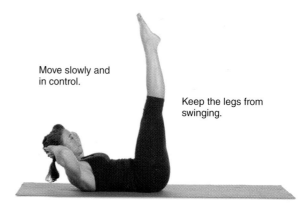

Move slowly and in control.

Keep the legs from swinging.

3 Exhale as you bring the legs back up above the hips. Repeat for 5 to 10 times.

Crisscross

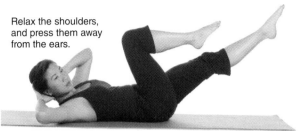

Relax the shoulders, and press them away from the ears.

Elbows stay out wide.

1 Lie on your back with one knee in tabletop position and the other stretched out at a 45-degree angle from the mat. Lift your head and shoulders, supporting your head with your hands, elbows out wide from the ears. Twist your upper torso toward the knee bent over the hips. Exhale in this position.

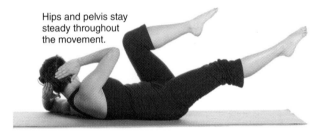

Hips and pelvis stay steady throughout the movement.

2 Inhale as you come on to your back through the center to switch sides. Exhale as you twist to the other side and switch your legs—the bent knee straightens as the straight leg draws in over the hip in tabletop position. Think of moving the rib cage toward the opposite hip instead of moving the elbow to the opposite knee. Repeat for 5 to 10 sets.

Contraindications
▶ Pain in, injuries to, or chronic conditions of the neck, torso, or shoulders

Focus
▶ Abdominals and muscles of the legs, arms, and back

Benefits
▶ Strengthens the abdominals
▶ Increases upper back flexibility
▶ Teaches core control
▶ Teaches breath and movement coordination

Teaser

Level

▶ Intermediate

Contraindications

▶ Pain in, injuries to, or chronic conditions of the torso

Focus

▶ Abdominals and muscles of the legs

Benefits

▶ Strengthens the abdominals and hip flexors
▶ Develops coordination and balance
▶ Teaches spinal articulation

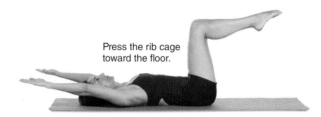

Press the rib cage toward the floor.

1 Lie on your back with the knees together and bent above the hips in tabletop position. Arms are straight and reaching over the head. If your shoulder area is tight, your arms might reach just above the mat.

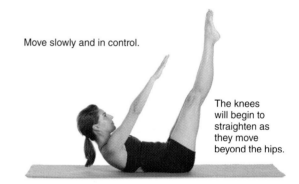

Move slowly and in control.

The knees will begin to straighten as they move beyond the hips.

2 Inhale as you lift the arms to the ceiling. Peel the head and shoulders off the mat. Begin to straighten the legs as you lift the head, neck, and shoulders.

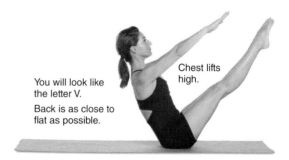

You will look like the letter V.

Back is as close to flat as possible.

Chest lifts high.

3 Exhale as you continue to roll up. Extend the legs at a 45-degree angle above the mat.

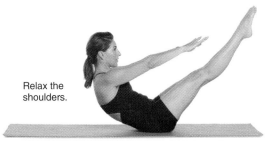

Relax the
shoulders.

Scoop the abdominals inward.

4 Inhale as you roll down the spine toward the floor. Keep the arms stretching forward.

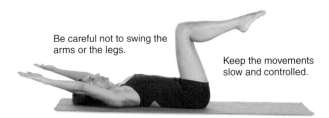

Be careful not to swing the
arms or the legs.

Keep the movements
slow and controlled.

5 Exhale as you continue to roll all the way down, bringing the arms above the head to the start position. Repeat from step 2 for 8 to 10 repetitions.

Shoulder Bridge

Level
▶ Intermediate

Contraindications
▶ Pain in, injuries to, or chronic conditions of the trunk or shoulders

Focus
▶ Muscles of the back, legs, and arms

Benefits
▶ Strengthens the back extensor muscles
▶ Strengthens the leg muscles, especially the hamstrings
▶ Increases core stability and strength

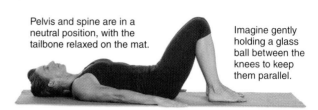

Pelvis and spine are in a neutral position, with the tailbone relaxed on the mat.

Imagine gently holding a glass ball between the knees to keep them parallel.

1 Lie on your back with the knees bent and heels in line with your sit bones. Hands are palms down on the mat by your sides. Inhale to prepare the body for the movement.

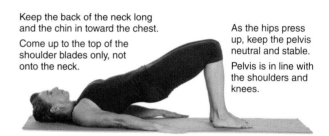

Keep the back of the neck long and the chin in toward the chest.

Come up to the top of the shoulder blades only, not onto the neck.

As the hips press up, keep the pelvis neutral and stable.

Pelvis is in line with the shoulders and knees.

2 Exhale as you press the hips up, creating a straight line with the knees, hips, and shoulders.

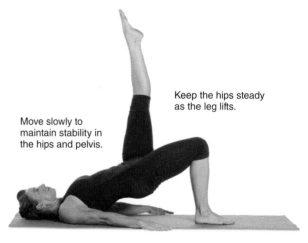

Keep the hips steady as the leg lifts.

Move slowly to maintain stability in the hips and pelvis.

3 Inhale as you lift one leg straight up and over the hip on that side, with the toes pointed to the ceiling.

Gentle Modification
If the hamstrings are tight, bend the lifted leg slightly so the pelvis does not tuck underneath.

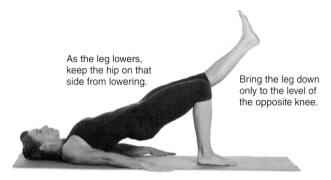

As the leg lowers, keep the hip on that side from lowering.

Bring the leg down only to the level of the opposite knee.

4 Exhale as you lower the lifted leg to the height of the hips, flexing the foot and bringing the toes toward the shins. Repeat steps 3 and 4 for five to eight times on one leg.

5 On the last repetition, bend the knee of the lifted leg and lower the foot to the floor. Keep the spine and pelvis neutral and stable as you move the legs. Relax the shoulders and neck. Stay in the bridge position. Switch legs and repeat steps 3 and 4 for five to eight times.

Rollover

Level

▶ Intermediate

Contraindications

▶ Pain in, injuries to, or chronic conditions of the torso or shoulders

Focus

▶ Abdominals and muscles of the back and scapulae

Benefits

▶ Strengthens the abdominals
▶ Increases lower back flexibility
▶ Teaches spinal articulation

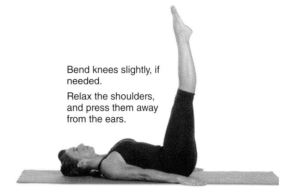

Bend knees slightly, if needed.

Relax the shoulders, and press them away from the ears.

1 Lie on the mat with your legs together and straight above your hips and your arms beside your body with the palms turned down. Inhale and pull the abdominals inward to ready the body.

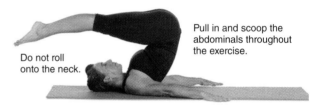

Pull in and scoop the abdominals throughout the exercise.

Do not roll onto the neck.

2 Exhale. Press into your hands, and roll the hips over the spine until the legs are above the head and parallel with the floor.

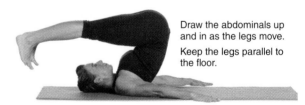

Draw the abdominals up and in as the legs move.

Keep the legs parallel to the floor.

3 Inhale as you separate the legs to sit-bone-distance apart and flex the feet.

4 Exhale and roll back down the spine until the legs are just above the hips. Inhale as you bring the legs together again and point the toes. Repeat from step 2 for four to six times. On the last repetition, do not bring the legs together again. Instead go to step 5 to reverse.

5 Keep the legs apart, back on the mat, legs just above hips. Inhale and point the toes. Exhale and roll the hips back over the spine until your legs are parallel to the floor. Inhale as you bring your legs together and flex the toes. Exhale and roll the spine back down to bring the legs back over the hips. Repeat four to six times.

Corkscrew

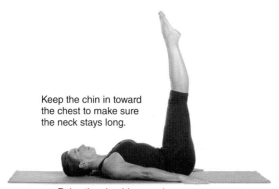

Keep the chin in toward the chest to make sure the neck stays long.

Relax the shoulders, and press them away from the ears.

1 Lie down on the mat with your legs together and straight above your hips. Arms are beside the body with the palms turned down.

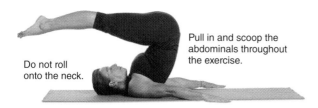

Do not roll onto the neck.

Pull in and scoop the abdominals throughout the exercise.

2 Inhale. Press into your hands, and roll the hips over the spine until the legs are above your head and parallel to the floor.

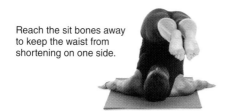

Reach the sit bones away to keep the waist from shortening on one side.

3 Exhale as you rotate the torso slightly to bring the legs to one side and roll down that side of the spine.

Level
▶ Advanced

Contraindications
▶ Pregnancy
▶ Pain in, injuries to, or chronic conditions of the neck, torso, or shoulders

Focus
▶ Abdominals and muscles of the back and shoulders

Benefits
▶ Stretches and massages the back muscles and the spine
▶ Activates and strengthens the abdominals
▶ Teaches shoulder stabilization
▶ Teaches core control

(continued)

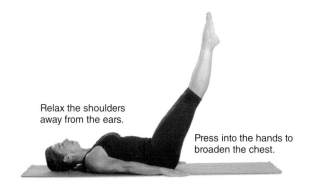

Relax the shoulders
away from the ears.

Press into the hands to
broaden the chest.

4 Continue to exhale as you bring the legs in a half circle around the tailbone and sacrum.

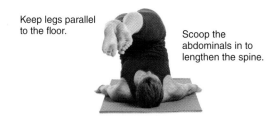

Keep legs parallel
to the floor.

Scoop the
abdominals in to
lengthen the spine.

5 Inhale as you roll up the other side of the spine and bring the legs back to the center. Repeat from step 3 for three to five sets.

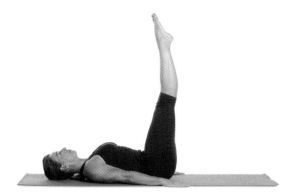

6 At the end of the last set, exhale and roll down the center of the spine to the start position.

Neck Pull

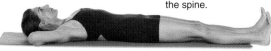

Relax the shoulders, and press them away from the ears.

Scoop the abdominals in, pressing them toward the spine.

1 Lie on the mat with the legs straight out, hip-distance apart, feet flexed to the ceiling, and the elbows bent and the hands supporting the head.

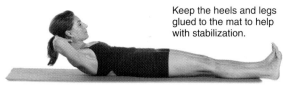

Keep the heels and legs glued to the mat to help with stabilization.

2 Inhale as you lift the head and then the spine off the mat.

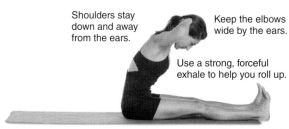

Shoulders stay down and away from the ears.

Keep the elbows wide by the ears.

Use a strong, forceful exhale to help you roll up.

Heels press into the ground.

3 Exhale as you continue to roll up until the torso sits on top of the sit bones and the upper body flexes forward and is parallel over the legs.

Level
▶ Advanced

Contraindications
▶ Pain in, injuries to, or chronic conditions of the neck or torso

Focus
▶ Abdominals and muscles of the back and scapulae

Benefits
▶ Strengthens the abdominals
▶ Increases back flexibility
▶ Teaches spinal articulation

(continued)

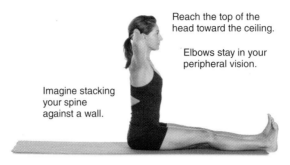

Reach the top of the
head toward the ceiling.

Elbows stay in your
peripheral vision.

Imagine stacking
your spine
against a wall.

4 Inhale as you restack the spine above the hips one vertebra at a time.

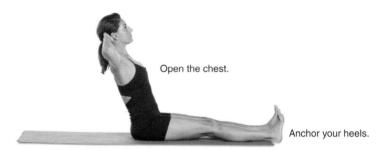

Open the chest.

Anchor your heels.

5 Exhale and hinge your torso back at the hips. Anchor your heels. Feel them reach away from your torso to ground the sit bones. Keep your elbows out wide to open the chest.

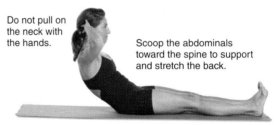

Do not pull on
the neck with
the hands.

Scoop the abdominals
toward the spine to support
and stretch the back.

Use the legs as an anchor.

6 Continue to exhale as you roll down one vertebra at a time until you are lying on the mat again. Repeat for three to five times.

Scissors

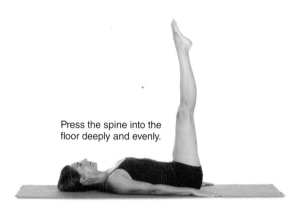

Press the spine into the floor deeply and evenly.

Level
▶ Advanced

Contraindications
▶ Pain in, injuries to, or chronic conditions of the neck, torso, wrists, or shoulders

Focus
▶ Abdominals and muscles of the back, arms, legs, and shoulders

1 Lie down on the mat with your legs together and straight above your hips, arms beside the body with the palms turned down. Inhale to prepare the body, and brace through the abdominals, scooping them inward.

Benefits
▶ Strengthens the abdominals
▶ Increases back flexibility
▶ Stretches the hamstrings and hip flexors

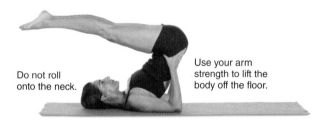

Do not roll onto the neck.

Use your arm strength to lift the body off the floor.

2 Exhale as you roll the back off the mat, bringing the legs up and over the buttocks. As you inhale, bring the hands underneath the hips, with the fingertips pointed outward and the wrists supporting the back and hips.

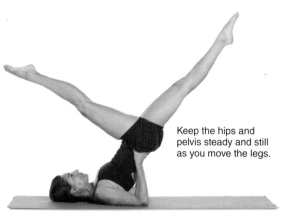

Keep the hips and pelvis steady and still as you move the legs.

3 Exhale as you scissor the legs; one leg moves over the head as the other leg moves toward the mat in the opposite direction.

(continued)

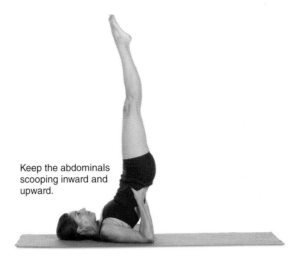

Keep the abdominals
scooping inward and
upward.

4 Inhale as you bring the legs back up over the hips.

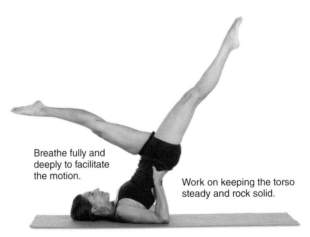

Breathe fully and
deeply to facilitate
the motion.

Work on keeping the torso
steady and rock solid.

5 Exhale as you scissor one leg over the head and the other one toward the mat. Repeat from step 3 for three to seven sets.

Bicycle

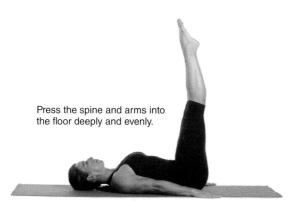

Press the spine and arms into the floor deeply and evenly.

Level
▶ Advanced

Contraindications
▶ Pain in, injuries to, or chronic conditions of the neck, torso, wrists, or shoulders

Focus
▶ Abdominals and muscles of the back, arms, legs, and shoulders

Benefits
▶ Strengthens the abdominals
▶ Increases back flexibility
▶ Stretches the hamstrings and hip flexors

1 Lie on the mat with your legs together and straight above your hips, arms beside the body with the palms turned down. Inhale to prepare the body, and brace through the abdominals, scooping them inward.

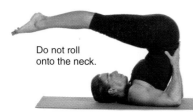

Do not roll onto the neck.

Use your arm strength to lift the body off the mat.

Open your chest by pressing your shoulders away from the ears.

2 Exhale as you roll the back off the mat, bringing the legs up and over the buttocks. As you inhale, bring the hands underneath the hips with the fingertips pointed outward and wrists supporting the back and hips.

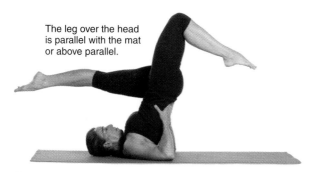

The leg over the head is parallel with the mat or above parallel.

3 Exhale as you hold one leg straight over the head and scissor the other leg over the body to bring it to a bent position, toes pointed toward the floor.

(continued)

Bicycle *(continued)*

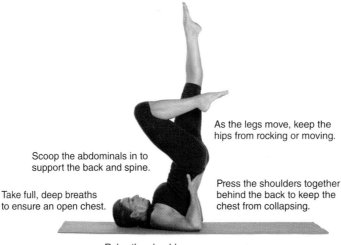

As the legs move, keep the
hips from rocking or moving.

Scoop the abdominals in to
support the back and spine.

Press the shoulders together
behind the back to keep the
chest from collapsing.

Take full, deep breaths
to ensure an open chest.

Relax the shoulders
away from the ears.

4 Inhale as you pull the bent knee over the hips as if riding a bicycle, and scissor the straight leg over the hips. Move the legs only as far as your flexibility allows and keep the movements slow and controlled.

5 Exhale as the bent knee straightens over the head and the straight leg bends and reaches toward the floor. Repeat this step for three to seven times in this direction. Switch directions, bicycling the legs in reverse three to seven times.

Jackknife

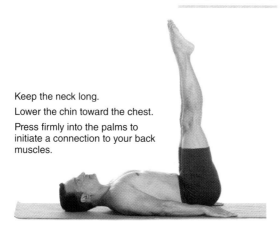

Keep the neck long.

Lower the chin toward the chest.

Press firmly into the palms to initiate a connection to your back muscles.

1 Lie on the mat with your legs together and straight above your hips, arms beside the body with the palms turned down. Inhale to prepare the body, and brace through the abdominals, scooping them inward.

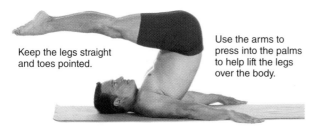

Keep the legs straight and toes pointed.

Use the arms to press into the palms to help lift the legs over the body.

2 Exhale as you roll the lower body off the mat. Bring the legs over the hips and the head until they are parallel to the mat.

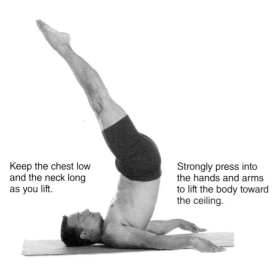

Keep the chest low and the neck long as you lift.

Strongly press into the hands and arms to lift the body toward the ceiling.

3 Inhale as you lift the legs toward the ceiling as much as your arms and core allow.

Level
▶ Advanced

Contraindications
▶ Pain in, injuries to, or chronic conditions of the neck, torso, or shoulders

Focus
▶ Abdominals and muscles of the back, arms, legs, and shoulders

Benefits
▶ Strengthens the abdominals
▶ Stretches the spine and back muscles
▶ Strengthens the arm muscles
▶ Teaches shoulder stability
▶ Teaches core control
▶ Teaches spinal articulation

(continued)

Jackknife *(continued)*

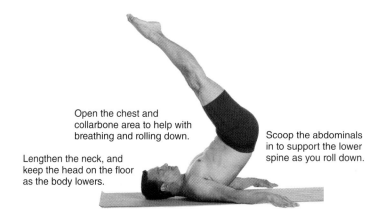

Open the chest and collarbone area to help with breathing and rolling down.

Lengthen the neck, and keep the head on the floor as the body lowers.

Scoop the abdominals in to support the lower spine as you roll down.

4 Exhale as you lower the body slowly and carefully one vertebra at a time.

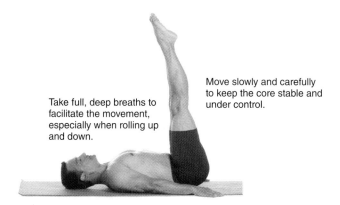

Take full, deep breaths to facilitate the movement, especially when rolling up and down.

Move slowly and carefully to keep the core stable and under control.

5 Finish exhaling in the same position in which you started, with the legs straight up above your hips and the spine flat along the mat, arms by your sides. Inhale to prepare for the next repetition or to finish. Repeat from step 2 for three repetitions.

Chapter 7

Seated Mat Exercises

Seated Pilates exercises focus on posture and core stabilization. Maintain an elongated torso and neck throughout these exercises, and relax the shoulders and scapulae. The chapter begins with a seated footwork series that heightens awareness of the movements of the feet, ankles, and lower legs. This awareness is critical for balance and stability when standing, and this series also promotes circulation and general awareness of overall posture.

Spine Stretch: Forward and Side

Level
▶ Beginner

Contraindications
▶ Pain in, injuries to, or chronic conditions of the spine or shoulders

Focus
▶ Abdominals and muscles of the back

Benefits
▶ Lengthens the spine (forward and side)
▶ Increases mobility of the shoulder joint
▶ Teaches correct sitting posture
▶ Strengthens and stabilizes the core and pelvis

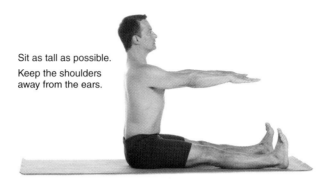

Sit as tall as possible.
Keep the shoulders away from the ears.

1 **Sit on the mat with the legs straight in front and sit-bone-distance apart. Arms are out in front of the shoulders, palms turned down. Put a prop under your hips if your hamstrings or lower back is tight.**

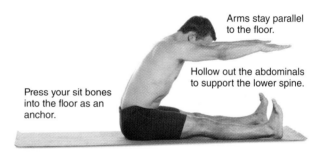

Arms stay parallel to the floor.

Hollow out the abdominals to support the lower spine.

Press your sit bones into the floor as an anchor.

2 **Inhale. Stretch the spine up and forward, creating a C-curve with the spine. As you stretch up and out, reach forward with the arms.**

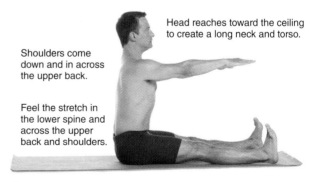

Head reaches toward the ceiling to create a long neck and torso.

Shoulders come down and in across the upper back.

Feel the stretch in the lower spine and across the upper back and shoulders.

3 **Exhale as you return to start position, spine tall and straight. Repeat from step 2 for five to eight times.**

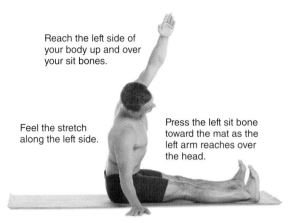

Reach the left side of your body up and over your sit bones.

Feel the stretch along the left side.

Press the left sit bone toward the mat as the left arm reaches over the head.

4 Inhale as you reach the right arm to the mat beside your right side and lift the left arm above your head and lean to the right, creating a C-curve with the right side of the body.

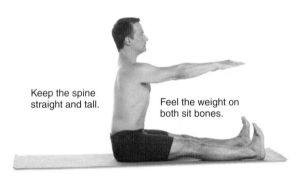

Keep the spine straight and tall.

Feel the weight on both sit bones.

5 Exhale as you return to a seated position, arms in front of the shoulders as in step 1.

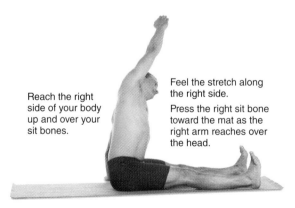

Feel the stretch along the right side.

Reach the right side of your body up and over your sit bones.

Press the right sit bone toward the mat as the right arm reaches over the head.

6 Inhale as you reach the left arm to the mat beside your left side and lift the right arm above your head and lean to the left, creating a C-curve with the left side of your body. Return to the seated position in step 5, and then repeat from step 4 for three to five sets on each side, alternating sides.

Mermaid

Level
▶ Beginner

Contraindications
▶ Pain in, injuries to, or conditions of the back, shoulders, wrists, or elbows

Focus
▶ Muscles of the arms, shoulders, and torso

Benefits
▶ Stretches each side of the waist
▶ Strengthens and stabilizes the wrists, hands, and shoulders

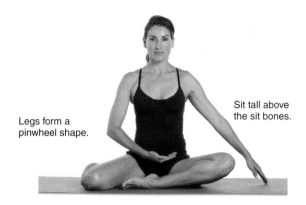

Legs form a pinwheel shape.

Sit tall above the sit bones.

1 **Sit on the mat with both legs bent and one foot touching the thigh of the other as the other foot points behind the body. One arm is straightened, with the palm or fingertips touching the mat beside the body, and the other is slightly bent and in the lap.**

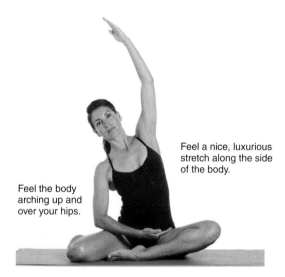

Feel the body arching up and over your hips.

Feel a nice, luxurious stretch along the side of the body.

2 **Inhale as you lift the arm on the mat over the head and in the direction of the legs as you bend the torso to that side.**

92

3 Exhale as you bring the hand back down beside the body with the palm down.

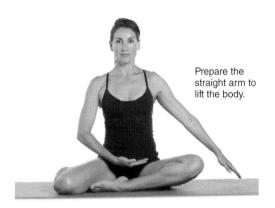

Prepare the straight arm to lift the body.

4 Inhale as you press into the hand on the mat and lift the hips as the free arm reaches over the head. Lift your head and eyes toward the lifted arm. Exhale as you sit down again. Repeat from step 2 for four to six repetitions.

Slightly press into the knees to stretch the hips forward and upward.

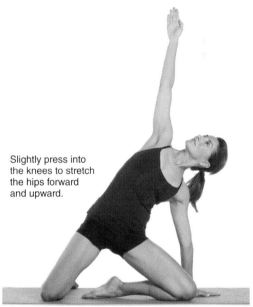

Knees stay on the floor.

Footwork Series

Level
▶ Beginner

Contraindications
▶ Pain in, injuries to, or chronic conditions of the spine, feet, or ankles

Focus
▶ Abdominals and muscles of the feet, legs, and back

Benefits
▶ Stretches the feet and improves articulation
▶ Mobilizes the ankle joint
▶ Teaches correct sitting posture
▶ Strengthens and stabilizes the core

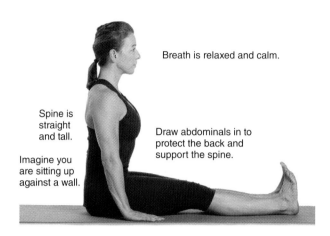

Breath is relaxed and calm.

Spine is straight and tall.

Imagine you are sitting up against a wall.

Draw abdominals in to protect the back and support the spine.

1 This exercise series warms up the feet, ankles, and lower legs. During these movements, keep the spine still and your breathing calm and focused. Begin by sitting with your legs straight in front of your hips, or use the gentle modification, if needed. Flex the feet up to the ceiling.

Gentle Modification
If your hamstrings or lower back is tight, place a bolster, block, or folded mat under your buttocks. If the hamstrings or lower back is still tight, bend the knees gently until the tension releases. Keep the knees bent throughout the exercises, if necessary.

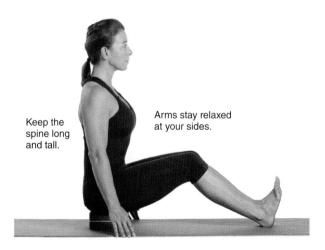

Keep the spine long and tall.

Arms stay relaxed at your sides.

Keep the knees and shins steady.

Imagine your feet are windshield wipers, moving side to side.

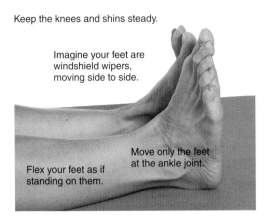

Flex your feet as if standing on them.

Move only the feet at the ankle joint.

2 Inhale as you move the feet to the right. Only the feet move.

Go slowly, using the breath to facilitate movement.

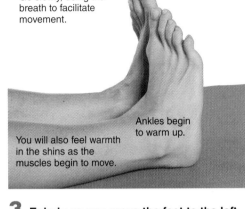

You will also feel warmth in the shins as the muscles begin to move.

Ankles begin to warm up.

3 Exhale as you move the feet to the left. Repeat steps 2 and 3 for 10 sets.

Toes reach away as far as possible to stretch the top of the foot.

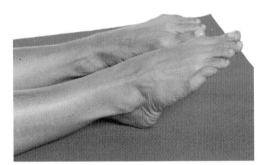

4 Inhale as you move both feet in a circular motion to the right from a flexed position. As you bring the foot around in the circle, point the toes away as far as possible to stretch the top of the foot.

Make the circle as large as possible, working the full range of motion for your feet.

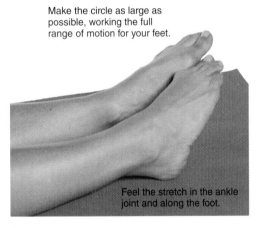

Feel the stretch in the ankle joint and along the foot.

5 Exhale and finish the half circle of the foot, bringing the feet up the left side of the ankle.

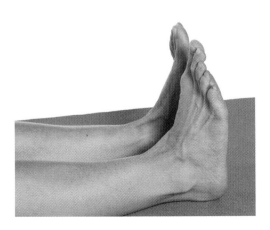

6 Finish the movement with the toes pointing to the ceiling, returning to the start position. When you finish each circle, strongly flex the foot to fully stretch the bottom of the foot, Achilles tendon, and calf. Repeat steps 4 and 5 for 10 repetitions. Repeat steps 4 and 5 again, starting the circle to the left for 10 repetitions.

(continued)

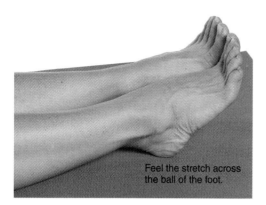

Feel the stretch across the ball of the foot.

Feel the stretch across the top of the foot and possibly the shin.

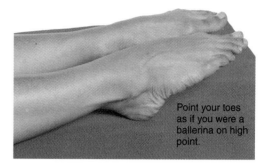

Point your toes as if you were a ballerina on high point.

7 Inhale as you press the ball of the foot away. Imagine you are wearing a pair of high heels or doing a calf raise. The ball of the foot presses away, but the toes point to the ceiling. Initially the range of motion might be small, but be patient. This range of motion will increase with time.

8 Exhale as you point the toes away from the body.

Reach up with the top of the head to keep the posture straight.

Remain tall and straight through the torso.

Pull in the abdominals to support the spine.

Keep the shoulders down and back.

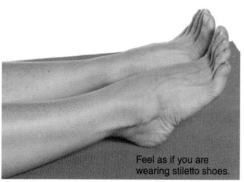

Feel as if you are wearing stiletto shoes.

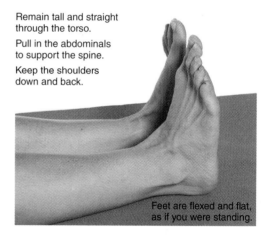

Feet are flexed and flat, as if you were standing.

9 Inhale as you pull just the toes up to the ceiling, pushing the ball of the foot away.

10 Exhale as you flex the toes back toward the shins. Repeat steps 6 through 10 for 5 to 10 repetitions.

Rolling Like a Ball

1 **Sit down. Lift your knees, and place your hands around the shins. Elbows are slightly bent and out to the sides.**

Look down between the knees.

Scoop the abdominals up and in to support the lower spine.

Balance between your sit bones and the tailbone.

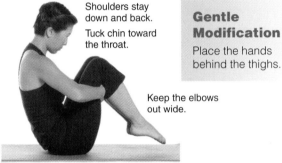

Level

▶ Beginner to intermediate

Contraindications

▶ Pain in, injuries to, or chronic conditions of the neck, shoulders, or lower back

Focus

▶ Abdominals and muscles of the scapulae

Benefits

▶ Strengthens the abdominals
▶ Increases lower back flexibility
▶ Improves shoulder stabilization
▶ Teaches core awareness and pelvis stability

Shoulders stay down and back.

Tuck chin toward the throat.

Gentle Modification

Place the hands behind the thighs.

Keep the elbows out wide.

2 **Inhale and roll back onto the upper back.**

Heels stay the same distance from the buttocks as you roll back.

Knees stay tight to the body.

Chin is in and head stays off the mat.

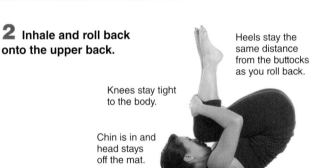

3 **Exhale and roll up to the start position. Find your balance between the sit bones and the tailbone for a second before executing the next repetition. Repeat for 8 to 10 times.**

Keep the shoulders away from the ears.

Contract and pull in the abdominals to stretch the lower back.

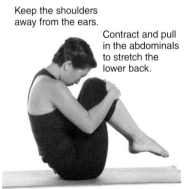

Side Bend

Level
▶ Intermediate

Contraindications
▶ Pain in, injuries to, and chronic conditions of the back, shoulders, wrists, or elbows

Focus
▶ Muscles of the arms, shoulders, wrists, and torso

Benefits
▶ Develops balance and coordination on one arm
▶ Stretches and works each side of the waist
▶ Strengthens the deep oblique muscles
▶ Strengthens and stabilizes the wrists, hands, and shoulders

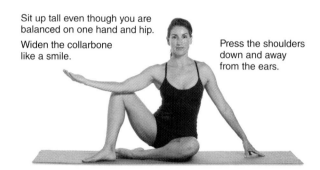

Sit up tall even though you are balanced on one hand and hip.

Widen the collarbone like a smile.

Press the shoulders down and away from the ears.

1 Sit on the mat on your left hip, with the left leg bent beside you and the right leg bent so the right foot is just in front of the left foot, with the foot flat and the knee pointed up. Place the right arm on the top of the right leg, with the palm turned toward the ceiling.

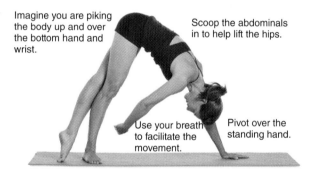

Imagine you are piking the body up and over the bottom hand and wrist.

Scoop the abdominals in to help lift the hips.

Use your breath to facilitate the movement.

Pivot over the standing hand.

2 Inhale as you lift the right arm and the hips and straighten the legs to lift the hips toward the ceiling and bring the head and right arm down. Balance on the left hand, left foot, and right toes. Your body will form an upside-down V with the hips in the air.

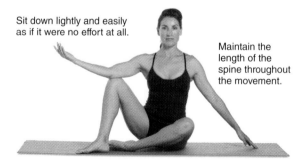

Sit down lightly and easily as if it were no effort at all.

Maintain the length of the spine throughout the movement.

3 Exhale as you lower the hips to the mat. Return to the start position by bending your knees and sitting down. Repeat three to five times. Switch sides and repeat three to five times.

Open Leg Rocker

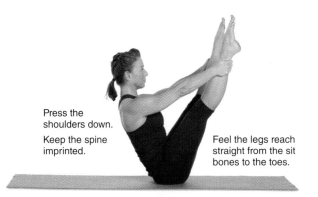

Press the shoulders down.

Keep the spine imprinted.

Feel the legs reach straight from the sit bones to the toes.

Level
▶ Intermediate

Contraindications
▶ Pain in, injuries to, or chronic conditions of the spine, shoulders, or back

Focus
▶ Abdominals and muscles of the back and scapulae

Benefits
▶ Improves scapular stability and strength
▶ Improves back flexibility
▶ Teaches coordination and balance of the torso
▶ Increases abdominal strength

1 Sit balanced between the sit bones and the tail-bone with the legs off the floor and stretched out in front of you, hands grasping each ankle. You will be seated in a V position. The upper body is upright and tall, and the abdominals are pulling inward and upward. Inhale to help yourself sit up tall and upright. Bend your knees slightly, if necessary, and grab the back of the upper legs instead of the ankles.

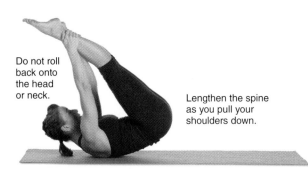

Do not roll back onto the head or neck.

Lengthen the spine as you pull your shoulders down.

2 Exhale as you roll back, tucking the chin to the chest and rounding the lower spine deeper. At the bottom of the rollback, inhale deeply.

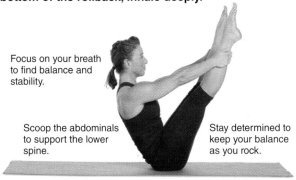

Focus on your breath to find balance and stability.

Scoop the abdominals to support the lower spine.

Stay determined to keep your balance as you rock.

3 Exhale as you roll up to a seated position, sitting on top of or just behind the sit bones and just in front of the tailbone. Repeat 5 to 10 times.

Spine Twist

Level
▶ Intermediate

Contraindications
▶ Pain in, injuries to, or chronic conditions of the spine, arms, or shoulders

Focus
▶ Abdominals and muscles of the back

Benefits
▶ Increases mobility and rotation of the spine
▶ Increases mobility of the shoulder joint
▶ Teaches correct sitting posture
▶ Strengthens and stabilizes the core and pelvis

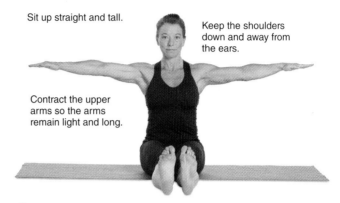

Sit up straight and tall.

Keep the shoulders down and away from the ears.

Contract the upper arms so the arms remain light and long.

1 **Sit on the mat with your legs together and straight in front of your hips. Lift your arms to shoulder level at your sides, palms turned down. Use the gentle modification (see Footwork Series, page 94), if needed, depending on your spine and hamstring flexibility.**

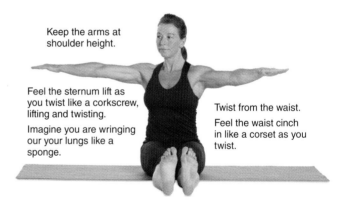

Keep the arms at shoulder height.

Feel the sternum lift as you twist like a corkscrew, lifting and twisting.

Imagine you are wringing our your lungs like a sponge.

Twist from the waist.

Feel the waist cinch in like a corset as you twist.

2 **While inhaling with a sniffing double breath, rotate the body to the right with a double pulse.**

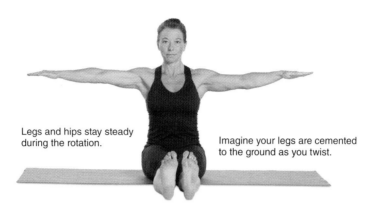

Legs and hips stay steady during the rotation.

Imagine your legs are cemented to the ground as you twist.

3 Exhale as you return to the start position with the torso upright, sitting on top of the hips, and the arms out to the sides.

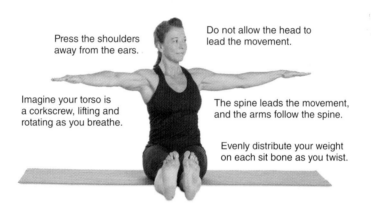

Press the shoulders away from the ears.

Do not allow the head to lead the movement.

Imagine your torso is a corkscrew, lifting and rotating as you breathe.

The spine leads the movement, and the arms follow the spine.

Evenly distribute your weight on each sit bone as you twist.

4 Inhale with a sniffing double breath as you rotate the body to the left with a double pulse. Return to the start position, and then repeat to the right. Repeat the sequence for four to six sets, alternating sides.

Saw

Level
▸ Intermediate

Contraindications
▸ Pain in, injuries to, or chronic conditions of the spine, arms, or shoulders

Focus
▸ Abdominals and muscles of the back

Benefits
▸ Increases mobility and rotation of the spine
▸ Increases mobility of the upper back and midback
▸ Teaches correct sitting posture
▸ Strengthens and stabilizes the core and pelvis

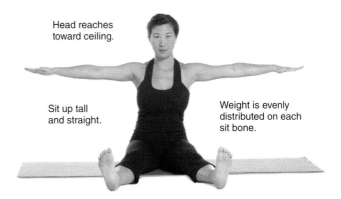

Head reaches toward ceiling.

Sit up tall and straight.

Weight is evenly distributed on each sit bone.

1 **Sit on the mat with your feet and legs a bit wider than shoulder-distance apart, feet flexed toward the ceiling, arms reaching out to the sides at shoulder height with the palms turned down.**

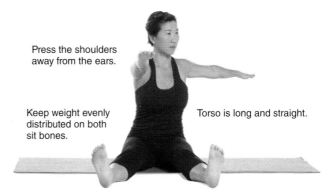

Press the shoulders away from the ears.

Keep weight evenly distributed on both sit bones.

Torso is long and straight.

2 Inhale as you rotate the upper body to the left, keeping the arms at shoulder height.

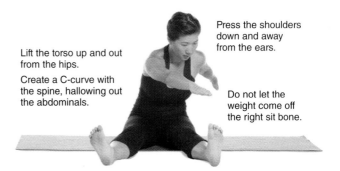

Lift the torso up and out from the hips.

Create a C-curve with the spine, hallowing out the abdominals.

Press the shoulders down and away from the ears.

Do not let the weight come off the right sit bone.

3 Exhale as you reach the right hand to the left foot and the left arm behind the body, twisting the torso to the left.

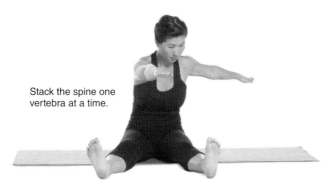

Stack the spine one vertebra at a time.

4 Inhale as you round up out of the stretch, keeping the upper body turned to the left.

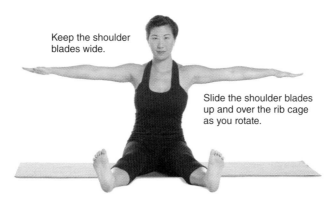

Keep the shoulder blades wide.

Slide the shoulder blades up and over the rib cage as you rotate.

5 Exhale as you return to the start position—seated upright with arms out to the sides. Repeat from step 2 for four to six sets, alternating sides.

Seal

Level
▶ Intermediate

Contraindications
▶ Pain in, injuries to, or chronic conditions of the spine, arms, legs, or shoulders

Focus
▶ Muscles of the spine, back, arms, shoulders, and legs

Benefits
▶ Stretches the spine and back muscles
▶ Increases the stability of the shoulder joint
▶ Increases coordination and balance

1 **Sit on the mat, balanced between the sit bones and tailbone. Bend the knees, and reach under the legs to grab the ankles with the hands. Knees are wide and toes are pointed toward one another. Spine is rounded and hollowed forward to support the lower spine and the back.**

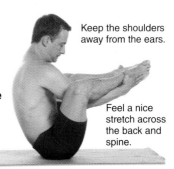

Keep the shoulders away from the ears.

Feel a nice stretch across the back and spine.

2 **Inhale as you roll back, keeping the head from touching the mat.**

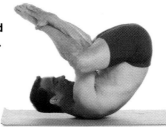

3 **Exhale. Stay rolled back as you clap the feet together three times.**

Maintain the hollowed-out position with the body.

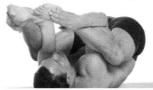

Use abdominal strength to support the back.

4 **Inhale as you roll up again, balancing in back of the sit bones. Exhale and clap the feet together three times, maintaining the hollowed-out position. Repeat from step 2 for 5 to 10 repetitions.**

Maintain the C-curve of the spine.

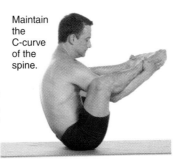

Boomerang

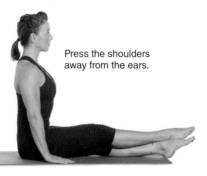

Feel light on the sit bones and long in the spine.

Imagine your back is pressed against a wall.

Press the shoulders away from the ears.

1 **Sit with the legs straight in front of the body, one leg crossed over the other, toes pointed and hands beside the body. Sit upright and straight. Inhale to prepare.**

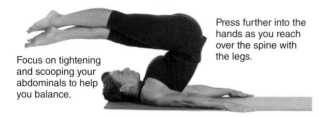

Keep the inner thighs close together.

Press your hands into the floor to keep the chest open wide.

2 **Exhale as you roll back (as in Rollover, page 78), bringing the straight legs over the head and torso until parallel to the floor behind the torso. Press the arms into the floor, and keep them wide as you roll over.**

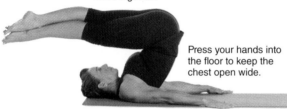

Press further into the hands as you reach over the spine with the legs.

Focus on tightening and scooping your abdominals to help you balance.

3 **Inhale as you uncross then recross the legs with the other leg in front.**

Level
▶ Advanced

Contraindications
▶ Pain in, injuries to, or chronic conditions of the spine, back, shoulders, or legs

Focus
▶ Abdominals and muscles of the back, legs, and arms

Benefits
▶ Strengthen the abdominals and back muscles
▶ Teaches coordination of movement with breath
▶ Teaches overall balance of the body during movement
▶ Strengthens and stretches the legs and arms

(continued)

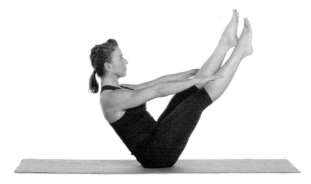

4 Exhale as you return to a seated position with the legs at a 45-degree angle, balancing as in Teaser (page 74) with the arms in front of the shoulders. Inhale as you circle the arms around and over the head until they are back in front of you.

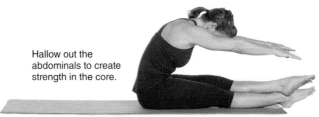

Hallow out the abdominals to create strength in the core.

Feel the lightness in your legs as you float them to the floor.

5 Exhale as you slowly lower the legs to the mat. Reach forward with the arms as you reach forward with the spine.

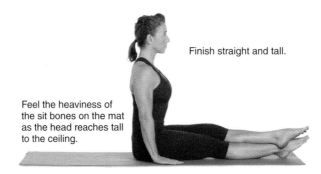

Finish straight and tall.

Feel the heaviness of the sit bones on the mat as the head reaches tall to the ceiling.

6 Inhale as you restack the spine and sit up tall again. Continue to inhale as you uncross then recross the legs. Repeat from step 2 for four to six times.

Chapter 8

Stability Ball Exercises

All the exercises in this chapter require the use of a stability ball. This ball is a fun accessory to bounce and stretch on and is also an excellent way to reinforce the most basic elements of Pilates training—core stabilization, core and full-body strengthening and flexibility, and balance. Exercises are organized into four categories: seated, prone, supine, and side lying.

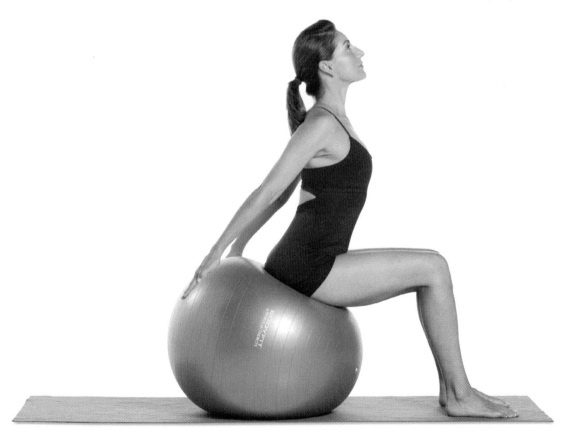

You will perform the first four stability ball exercises while seated on the stability ball, with the feet on the floor and the butt on the ball itself (figure 8.1). Your spine should be straight up and down as if up against a wall, with the shoulders relaxed and down away from the ears and the eyes straight ahead. Feet and knees are hip-distance apart, with the knees bent at a 90-degree angle. Arms relax beside you by the hips and under the shoulders. You should be propped up toward the front edge of the ball and not toward the back end or middle of the ball.

For the supine series, you will perform the exercises while lying on your back on the mat. The ball will be in the hands or between the feet. The specifics for placing the spine in the correct position (neutral, supported neutral, and imprint) are discussed in chapter 6 (pages 58-59). Please review that section before continuing with the supine stability ball exercises.

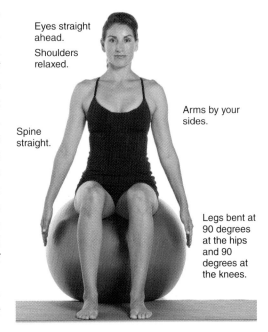

Eyes straight ahead.
Shoulders relaxed.

Spine straight.

Arms by your sides.

Legs bent at 90 degrees at the hips and 90 degrees at the knees.

Figure 8.1 Seated position on the stability ball.

All the prone stability ball exercises are done as you face the mat with the stability ball underneath your body (figure 8.2), either at the hips or somewhere on the legs. The spine and back should be in a neutral position. Lie facedown over the ball, and roll forward until the hands are on the mat in front of the ball and the hips are on

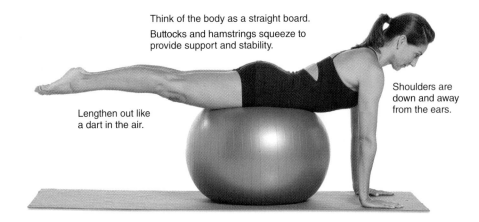

Think of the body as a straight board.
Buttocks and hamstrings squeeze to provide support and stability.

Lengthen out like a dart in the air.

Shoulders are down and away from the ears.

Figure 8.2 Prone position on the stability ball.

the ball in the center, with the legs stretched straight out from the hips and the toes pointed away from the body.

For the side-lying stability ball exercises, you will drape the side of your body over the stability ball. There are two basic positions for the side-lying series—a modified easier version and a more challenging balanced version.

For the easier version (figure 8.3), lie on your right side with the ball under the right rib cage. Bend the right leg, and place that knee on the mat at a 45-degree angle from the hip. Drape your upper body over the ball, and place your right hand on the mat on the other side of the ball. The left leg is straight out from the hip or just below and hovering above the floor, ready to be worked. The left hand is behind the head, with the elbow bent and pointed toward the ceiling.

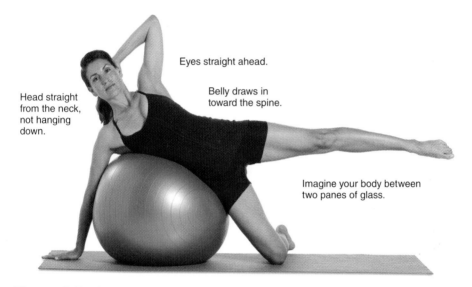

Eyes straight ahead.

Belly draws in toward the spine.

Head straight from the neck, not hanging down.

Imagine your body between two panes of glass.

Figure 8.3 Side-lying position on the stability ball: easier version.

For a more challenging version (figure 8.4), lie on your right side with the ball under the right hip. Stretch out both legs from the hips. With the legs stacked, drape your upper body from the waist up over the ball, and place your right hand on the mat on the other side of the ball. The legs are straight out, ready to be worked. The top hand is behind the head, with the elbow bent and pointed to the ceiling.

For the side-lying exercises, you can perform all exercises as a series or each as an individual exercise. Whether you do them individually or as a series, they do need to be done on both sides of the body to create balance and symmetry. You may choose to change from side to side for each exercise or perform each exercise on one side of the body, switch sides, and repeat each exercise on the other side.

The size and feel of the ball will vary depending on how much air is in the ball. A basic guideline for determining the correct size of the ball is to sit on it with your feet on the ground. You want your thighs to be straight out from your hips and parallel to the floor. If your knees are bent and your feet flat on the floor, your body creates a 90-degree angle at the hip and a 90-degree angle at the knee (figure 8.1). If the ball

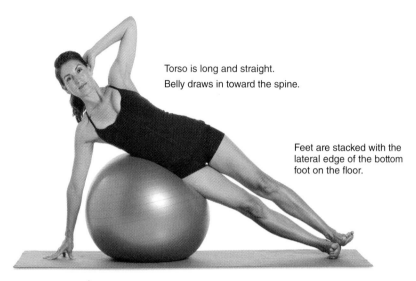

Torso is long and straight.
Belly draws in toward the spine.

Feet are stacked with the lateral edge of the bottom foot on the floor.

Figure 8.4 Side-lying position on the stability ball: challenging version.

is too full, it will not provide the correct amount of rebound when you push or sit on it, and it will probably not be stable enough to be effective. If the ball is too small, you will not feel stable when you sit on it, and your core will not be activated. The following is a general guideline for the proper ball size according to your height:

- ▶ Less than 5 feet (153 cm) tall: 45 cm
- ▶ 5 feet to 5 feet, 7 inches (170 cm): 55 cm
- ▶ 5 feet, 7 inches to 6 feet, 2 inches (188 cm): 65 cm
- ▶ More than 6 feet, 2 inches: 75 cm

Please keep in mind that this is only a general guideline and that the ball size depends more on the length of your legs than your height. Go back to the rule that the legs should be at a 90-degree angle, with your thighs parallel to the floor and the hips the same height as the knees.

One other point about working with the stability ball is that it does have a tendency to wander. When working with the ball, please pay attention to where the ball is at all times. When standing or sitting on the ball, touch the ball with one or both hands or a finger at all times to stay aware of where the ball is and where it might be going. You will also want to work in a room where there is no furniture in the way or nearby and where there is plenty of room between the ball and the wall so as to prevent injury.

The first few exercises are excellent for aerobic conditioning because they increase the heart rate. Then we will move into some stretches followed by the core conditioning exercises.

Bouncing in Place

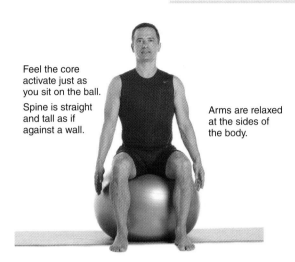

Feel the core activate just as you sit on the ball.

Spine is straight and tall as if against a wall.

Arms are relaxed at the sides of the body.

1 Sit on the ball with the feet directly in front of the hips and the heels directly below the knees.

Level
▶ Beginner

Contraindications
▶ Pain in, injuries to, or chronic conditions of the lower back, knees, or ankles

Focus
▶ Abdominals
▶ Overall conditioning

Benefits
▶ Trains balance and coordination of the core and spine
▶ Strengthens the legs and improves awareness
▶ Develops overall balance and coordination
▶ Builds aerobic capacity

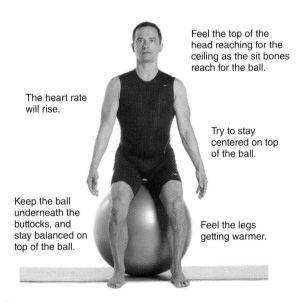

Feel the top of the head reaching for the ceiling as the sit bones reach for the ball.

The heart rate will rise.

Try to stay centered on top of the ball.

Keep the ball underneath the buttocks, and stay balanced on top of the ball.

Feel the legs getting warmer.

2 Push down into the heels and lift the buttocks, and begin bouncing on the ball. Create lift by pressing down into the heels and activating the hamstrings as well as the core, making your body light so you bounce easily and effortlessly. Breathe in through the nose and out through the mouth with ease, taking full and complete breaths. Repeat 30 to 50 times or for approximately 2 minutes.

Bouncing While Kicking

Level
▶ Beginner

Contraindications
▶ Injuries to, pain in, or chronic conditions of the lower back, knees, or ankles

Focus
▶ Abdominals and muscles of the legs
▶ Overall conditioning

Benefits
▶ Improves balance and coordination of the core and spine
▶ Strengthens the legs and improves awareness
▶ Develops overall balance and coordination
▶ Builds aerobic capacity

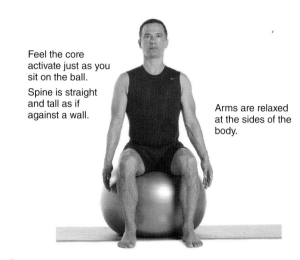

Feel the core activate just as you sit on the ball.

Spine is straight and tall as if against a wall.

Arms are relaxed at the sides of the body.

1 Sit on the ball with the feet directly in front of the hips and the heels directly below the knees. Arms are at your sides, hands lightly touching the ball for support.

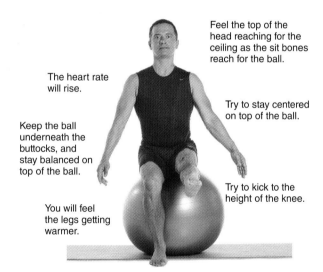

Feel the top of the head reaching for the ceiling as the sit bones reach for the ball.

The heart rate will rise.

Try to stay centered on top of the ball.

Keep the ball underneath the buttocks, and stay balanced on top of the ball.

Try to kick to the height of the knee.

You will feel the legs getting warmer.

2 Push down into the heels, and feel the buttocks squeeze together as you bounce up on the ball while kicking one leg in front of you. Switch legs on each bounce. Repeat for 30 to 50 times or for 1 to 2 minutes.

Challenge
Once you have built up your core strength and confidence, try bouncing with the arms crossed in front of the body. If you lose your balance, bring the hands down to touch the ball.

Bouncing With Arm Raised

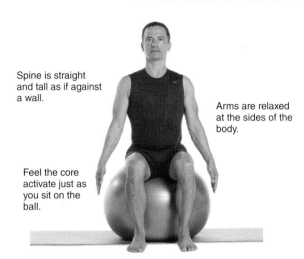

Spine is straight and tall as if against a wall.

Arms are relaxed at the sides of the body.

Feel the core activate just as you sit on the ball.

1 Sit on the ball with the feet directly in front of the hips and the heels directly below the knees. Arms are at your sides, hands lightly touching the ball for support.

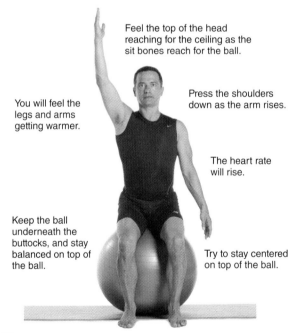

Feel the top of the head reaching for the ceiling as the sit bones reach for the ball.

You will feel the legs and arms getting warmer.

Press the shoulders down as the arm rises.

The heart rate will rise.

Keep the ball underneath the buttocks, and stay balanced on top of the ball.

Try to stay centered on top of the ball.

2 Push down with the heels, and feel the hips and buttocks tighten as you bounce up on the ball while raising one arm over the head. Switch arms on each bounce. Repeat for 30 to 50 times or for 1 to 2 minutes.

Level
▶ Beginner

Contraindications
▶ Injuries to, pain in, or chronic conditions of the lower back, knees, ankles, or arms

Focus
▶ Abdominals and muscles of the legs and arms
▶ Overall conditioning

Benefits
▶ Improves balance and coordination of the core and spine
▶ Strengthens the legs and improves awareness
▶ Develops overall balance and coordination
▶ Builds aerobic capacity
▶ Builds coordination of arms and legs moving together

Challenge
Try keeping one arm up for two bounces and then switching arms.

Pelvic Clock With Stretching on the Ball

Level
► Beginner

Contraindications
► Injuries to, pain in, or chronic conditions of the lower back, knees, ankles, or arms

Focus
► Abdominals, spine, and muscles of the arms and trunk

Benefits
► Promotes balance and coordination of the core and spine
► Develops overall balance and coordination
► Improves spinal articulation and warming
► Stretches and lengthens the arms

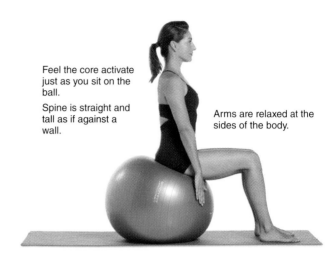

Feel the core activate just as you sit on the ball.

Spine is straight and tall as if against a wall.

Arms are relaxed at the sides of the body.

1 Sit on the ball with the feet directly in front of the hips and the heels directly below the knees. Arms are at your sides, hands lightly touching the ball for support.

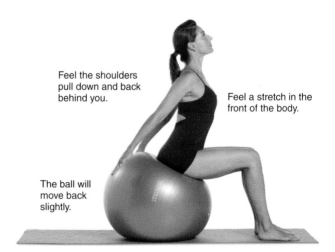

Feel the shoulders pull down and back behind you.

Feel a stretch in the front of the body.

The ball will move back slightly.

2 Inhale as you lift the chest and sternum and look to the upper corner of the room. Reach the arms behind you, and move the ball so the tailbone points up behind you.

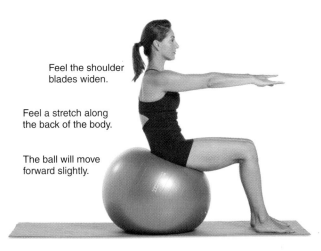

Feel the shoulder blades widen.

Feel a stretch along the back of the body.

The ball will move forward slightly.

3 Exhale as you push back with your legs. Round the spine forward by tucking the tailbone underneath you as you bring the arms in front of the body and stretch forward with the hands.

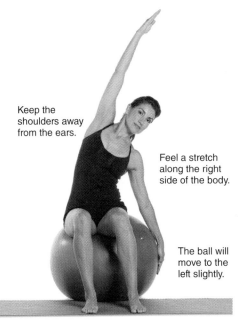

Keep the shoulders away from the ears.

Feel a stretch along the right side of the body.

The ball will move to the left slightly.

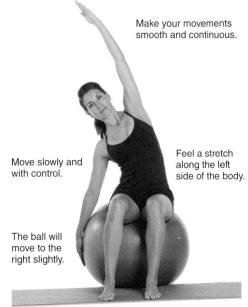

Make your movements smooth and continuous.

Move slowly and with control.

Feel a stretch along the left side of the body.

The ball will move to the right slightly.

4 Inhale as you lift the right arm over the head and contract the left side of your body to stretch the right side. Exhale and return to the start position.

5 Inhale as you lift the left arm over the head and contract the right side of your body to stretch the left side. Exhale and return to the start position. Repeat steps 2 through 5 for four to six repetitions.

Roll-Up Variations With the Ball

Level

▶ Beginner to intermediate

Contraindications

▶ Injuries to, pain in, or chronic conditions of the spine, neck, back, or shoulders

Focus

▶ Abdominals and muscles of the back, arms, and shoulders

Benefits

▶ Strengthens the abdominals
▶ Increases lower back flexibility
▶ Teaches spinal articulation
▶ Builds upper body coordination and strength

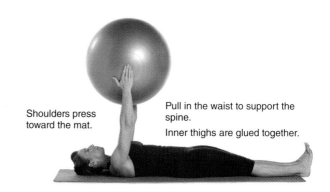

Shoulders press toward the mat.

Pull in the waist to support the spine.

Inner thighs are glued together.

1 Lie down on the mat with the stability ball in your hands and the arms extended above the shoulders. Legs are straight on the mat with the inner thighs together and the feet flexed toward the ceiling.

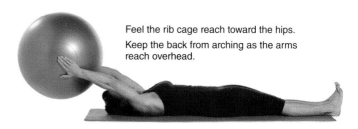

Feel the rib cage reach toward the hips.

Keep the back from arching as the arms reach overhead.

2 Inhale as you lift the ball over the head, keeping the arms straight.

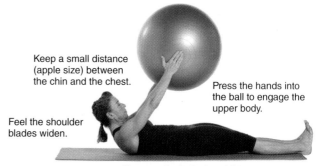

Keep a small distance (apple size) between the chin and the chest.

Press the hands into the ball to engage the upper body.

Feel the shoulder blades widen.

Squeeze the buttocks a bit to assist in lifting the upper body.

3 Exhale as you lift the ball up and forward and begin to roll up. As you roll up, lift the head first and then continue to roll up.

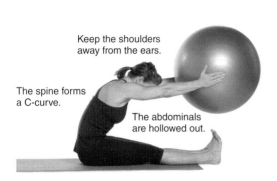

Keep the shoulders away from the ears.

The spine forms a C-curve.

The abdominals are hollowed out.

4 Finish the exhale with the body curved forward and the ball reaching over your legs, parallel to the floor.

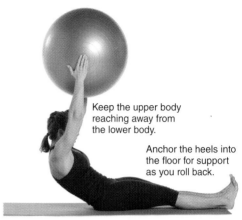

Keep the upper body reaching away from the lower body.

Anchor the heels into the floor for support as you roll back.

Squeeze the inner thighs together.

5 Inhale as you begin to roll back down, bringing the ball up toward the ears. Continue to inhale and roll down the spine one vertebra at a time until the head touches the mat and the ball is over the head.

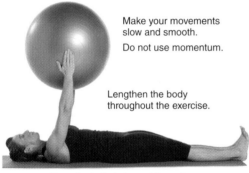

Make your movements slow and smooth.

Do not use momentum.

Lengthen the body throughout the exercise.

Draw the belly in toward the spine.

6 Exhale as you bring the ball up and over the shoulders, keeping the rest of the body still. Repeat steps 2 through 6 for four to six repetitions.

Challenge

Follow steps 2 through 6, except that when rolling down (step 5), roll slightly to one side on the way down, and switch to the other side the next time down.

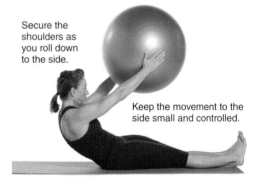

Secure the shoulders as you roll down to the side.

Keep the movement to the side small and controlled.

Rollover Pass the Ball

Level
▶ Intermediate to advanced

Contraindications
▶ Injuries to, pain in, or chronic conditions of the spine, neck, back, or shoulders

Focus
▶ Abdominals and muscles of the back, arms, and shoulders

Benefits
▶ Strengthens the abdominals
▶ Increases lower and upper back flexibility
▶ Teaches spinal articulation
▶ Builds upper body coordination and strength

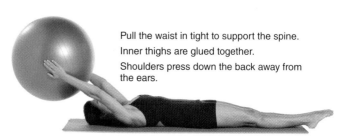

Pull the waist in tight to support the spine.

Inner thighs are glued together.

Shoulders press down the back away from the ears.

1 Lie on the mat with the ball in your hands and the arms extended over the head. Legs are extended straight on the mat, with the inner thighs together and the feet pointed away from the torso. Prepare with a deep inhale.

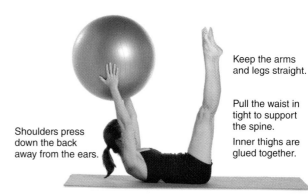

Shoulders press down the back away from the ears.

Keep the arms and legs straight.

Pull the waist in tight to support the spine.

Inner thighs are glued together.

2 Exhale as you lift the ball over the head and shoulders and the feet off the mat toward the ceiling.

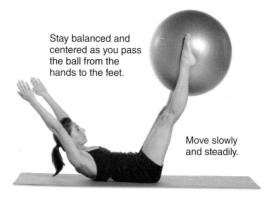

Stay balanced and centered as you pass the ball from the hands to the feet.

Move slowly and steadily.

3 Inhale as you pass the ball from the hands to between the ankles.

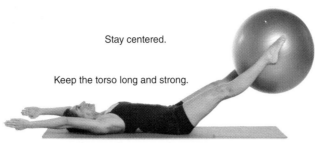

Stay centered.

Keep the torso long and strong.

Contract the core as the
legs and arms lower.

4 Exhale as you lower the legs toward the mat and roll down the upper body
with the arms as close to the ears as possible. Continue to exhale as you lower
the feet, head, and arms to the mat at the same time. Repeat from step 1 for 5 to 10
repetitions.

Modification

When lowering the upper body, keep the arms in front of the
chest and bend the knees slightly.

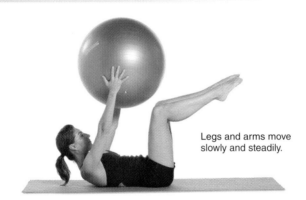

Legs and arms move
slowly and steadily.

Bridging Variations on the Ball

Level
▶ Beginner to intermediate

Contraindications
▶ Injuries to, pain in, or chronic conditions of the spine, neck, back, or shoulders

Focus
▶ Abdominals and muscles of the back, buttocks, arms, and shoulders

Benefits
▶ Strengthens the hamstrings, buttocks, abdominals, and back
▶ Teaches spinal articulation
▶ Builds upper and lower body coordination and strength

Knees and hips form a 90-degree angle.

Arms press firmly into the mat to open the chest and provide support for the lift.

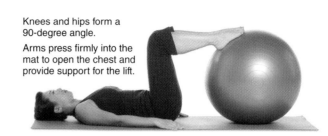

1 Lie on your back with your knees bent at 90 degrees above the hips and feet straight out from your knees and flat on the ball. Inhale to prepare.

Press feet deeply into the ball to avoid extra ball movement.

Keep the collarbone area open and wide.

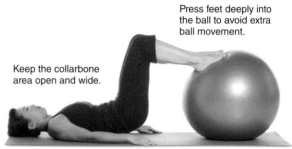

Feel the spine lift off the floor one vertebra at a time.

2 Exhale as you begin to curl the tailbone under, and lift the hips slowly toward a bridge position.

Think long and strong.

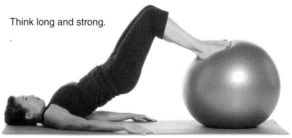

Press the hands to the mat to open the chest wide.

3 Inhale at the top of the bridge movement. Send the breath down the tops of the legs, and feel the length and strength of the movement.

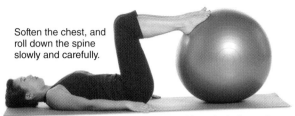

Soften the chest, and roll down the spine slowly and carefully.

Press the knees and inner thighs together.

Keep the ball steady under the feet.

4 **Exhale as you slowly roll down the spine toward the mat. Repeat for 5 to 10 repetitions.**

Challenge 1

For the straight-leg bridge variation, lie on the mat with the legs extended and the calves on the ball, legs pressed together for support. Follow steps 1 through 4 with straight legs for 5 to 10 repetitions. It is more of a challenge when the legs are straight. Feel connected through the core as you lift and lower the body into and out of the bridge position.

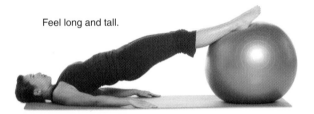

Feel long and tall.

Challenge 2

For the one-leg bridge variation, follow steps 1 and 2 with straight legs. At the top of the bridge, as you inhale, lift one leg above the hips and then exhale to lower the foot back to the ball, staying in the bridge position. Repeat, alternating legs for four to six sets. After your last set, inhale at the top of the lift and then exhale to lower the spine down to the mat.

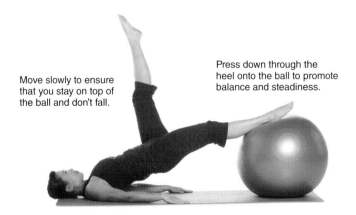

Move slowly to ensure that you stay on top of the ball and don't fall.

Press down through the heel onto the ball to promote balance and steadiness.

Hundred With the Ball

Level

▶ Beginner to intermediate

Contraindications

▶ Injuries to, pain in, or chronic conditions of the torso, neck, or shoulders

Focus

▶ Abdominals and muscles of the back, arms, legs, and shoulders

Benefits

▶ Strengthens the abdominals
▶ Teaches correct breathing with abdominal engagement
▶ Increases upper back flexibility
▶ Builds coordination of arm movement with breath

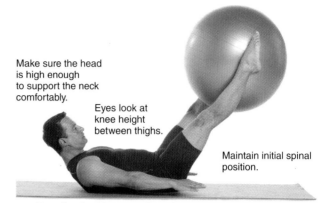

Make sure the head is high enough to support the neck comfortably.

Eyes look at knee height between thighs.

Maintain initial spinal position.

Keep the shoulders away from the ears.

1 Lie on your back with the ball between the ankles and the legs straight out from the hips at a 45-degree angle. Lift the head so the eyes look between the thighs. Arms are straight out from the shoulders and hovering just above the mat with the palms turned down.

2 Inhale as you pulse the arms for five counts (approximately 5 seconds). Keep the upper body still.

3 Exhale as you pulse the arms for five counts (approximately 5 seconds). Repeat for 10 repetitions or breaths.

Single-Leg Stretch With the Ball

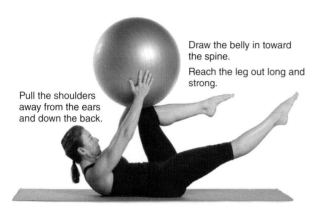

Pull the shoulders away from the ears and down the back.

Draw the belly in toward the spine.

Reach the leg out long and strong.

Level
▶ Beginner to intermediate

Contraindications
▶ Injuries to, pain in, or chronic conditions of the neck, torso, or shoulders

Focus
▶ Abdominals and muscles of the back, arms, and shoulders

Benefits
▶ Strengthens the abdominals
▶ Teaches spinal articulation
▶ Builds coordination of arm and leg movement with breath

1 Lie on your back with one knee bent toward the chest and the other leg out at a 45-degree angle to the mat. Hold the stability ball in your hands above the shin of the bent knee as you lift the head, neck, and shoulders.

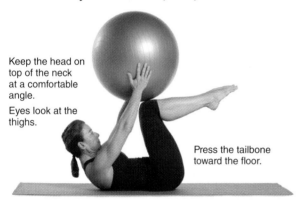

Keep the head on top of the neck at a comfortable angle.

Eyes look at the thighs.

Press the tailbone toward the floor.

2 Inhale as you draw the straight leg toward the chest over the hips.

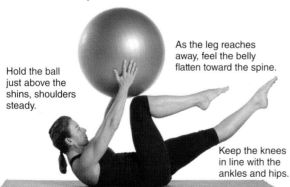

Hold the ball just above the shins, shoulders steady.

As the leg reaches away, feel the belly flatten toward the spine.

Keep the knees in line with the ankles and hips.

3 Exhale as you extend the other leg at a 45-degree angle to the mat. Repeat steps 2 and 3 for 10 sets. Each time the knees pass each other, they should touch lightly.

Double-Leg Stretch With the Ball

Level

▶ Beginner to intermediate

Contraindications

▶ Injuries to, pain in, or chronic conditions of the torso, neck, or shoulders

Focus

▶ Abdominals and muscles of the back, arms, and shoulders

Benefits

▶ Strengthens the abdominals
▶ Teaches spinal articulation
▶ Increases upper back flexibility
▶ Builds coordination of arm and leg movement with breath

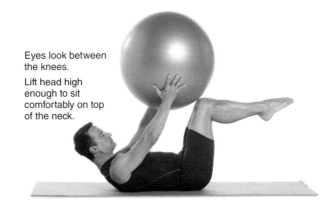

Eyes look between the knees.

Lift head high enough to sit comfortably on top of the neck.

1 Lie on your back with both knees bent in toward the chest. Hold the ball in your hands over the shins, with the head lifted toward the knees.

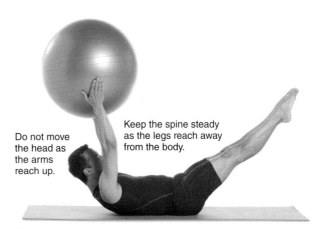

Do not move the head as the arms reach up.

Keep the spine steady as the legs reach away from the body.

2 Inhale as you bring the arms toward the ears over the head and reach the legs out straight at a 45-degree angle to the mat.

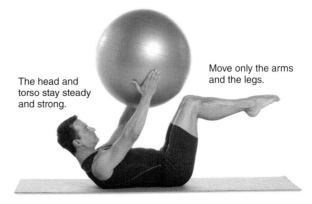

The head and torso stay steady and strong.

Move only the arms and the legs.

3 Exhale as you draw the knees into the chest and lower the arms, bringing the ball back over the shins.

Single Straight-Leg Stretch With the Ball

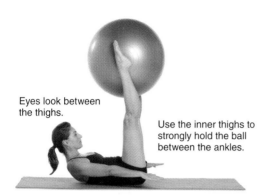

Eyes look between the thighs.

Use the inner thighs to strongly hold the ball between the ankles.

Level
▶ Intermediate

Contraindications
▶ Injuries to, pain in, or chronic conditions of the torso, neck, or shoulders

Focus
▶ Abdominals and muscles of the back, arms, legs, and shoulders

Benefits
▶ Strengthens the abdominals
▶ Increases upper back and hamstring flexibility
▶ Teaches spinal articulation
▶ Builds coordination of arm and leg movement with breath

1 Lie on your back. Place the ball between your ankles, and reach your legs up toward the ceiling. Reach the arms out straight and just above the mat, palms turned down as you lift the head, neck, and shoulders off the mat.

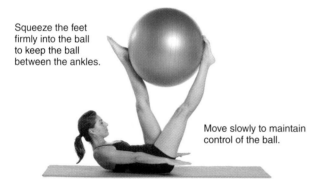

Squeeze the feet firmly into the ball to keep the ball between the ankles.

Move slowly to maintain control of the ball.

2 Inhale with a double breath as you rotate the legs and bring the ball to the side. One leg comes closer to your head. As you inhale and turn the legs, pulse your arms down for two breaths.

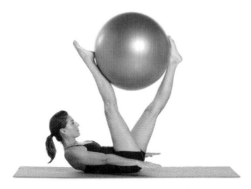

3 Exhale as you return the legs to the start position, holding the ball between the ankles. Inhale with another double breath, and rotate the legs to the other side. Repeat steps 2 and 3, alternating sides, for 10 sets.

Double Straight-Leg Stretch With the Ball

Level

▶ Intermediate

Contraindications

▶ Injuries to, pain in, or chronic conditions of the torso, neck, or shoulders

Focus

▶ Abdominals and muscles of the back, arms, legs, and shoulders

Benefits

▶ Strengthens the abdominals
▶ Increases upper back flexibility
▶ Teaches core control
▶ Builds coordination of arm and leg movement with breath

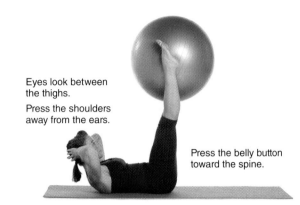

Eyes look between the thighs.

Press the shoulders away from the ears.

Press the belly button toward the spine.

1 Lie on your back with your legs in the air toward the ceiling. Place the ball between your ankles. Lift your head, placing your hands behind the head to support the neck, elbows bent. Inhale to prepare the body.

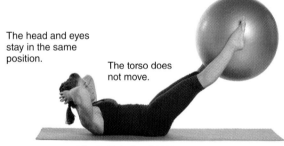

The head and eyes stay in the same position.

The torso does not move.

The belly button keeps pressing toward the spine.

2 Exhale as you lower the legs to a 45-degree angle from the mat.

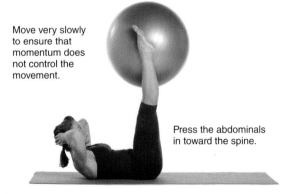

Move very slowly to ensure that momentum does not control the movement.

Press the abdominals in toward the spine.

3 Inhale as you lift the legs to a 90-degree position, with the feet directly above the hips and sit bones.

Crisscross With the Ball

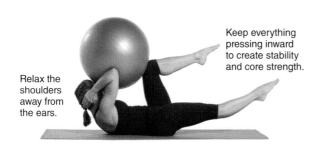

Relax the shoulders away from the ears.

Keep everything pressing inward to create stability and core strength.

Level
▶ Intermediate

Contraindications
▶ Injuries to, pain in, or chronic conditions of the torso, neck, or shoulders

Focus
▶ Abdominals and muscles of the back, arms, and shoulders

1 Lie on the mat with the knees bent and the ball balanced between both elbows, the left knee, and the forehead. Reach the right leg straight and long away from the torso, and hover it just above the mat. Exhale and press everything inward to support the back and torso as you twist the upper body toward the left knee.

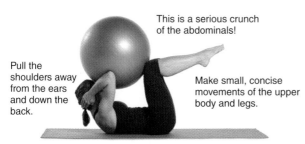

Pull the shoulders away from the ears and down the back.

This is a serious crunch of the abdominals!

Make small, concise movements of the upper body and legs.

Benefits
▶ Strengthens the abdominals
▶ Increases upper back flexibility
▶ Teaches core control
▶ Builds coordination of arm and leg movement with breath

2 Inhale as you bring the right knee to the ball so that both elbows and knees are touching the ball. The upper body lifts toward the centerline of the knees and up toward the ball.

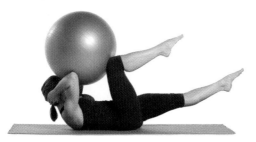

3 Exhale as you press away the left leg, holding the ball between the right knee and both elbows. As you exhale and press away the left leg, the upper body lifts higher and rotates slightly toward the right knee. Repeat from step 2, alternating legs for 10 sets.

Swan on the Ball

Level
▶ Intermediate

Contraindications
▶ Injuries to, chronic conditions of, or pain in the back, spine, shoulders, arms, or wrists

Focus
▶ Muscles of the arms, back, and legs

Benefits
▶ Strengthens the hamstrings and buttocks
▶ Strengthens the back muscles
▶ Creates core awareness
▶ Builds coordination

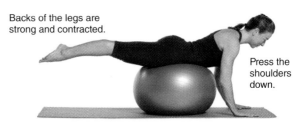

Backs of the legs are strong and contracted.

Press the shoulders down.

1 Lie on the stability ball with the hips on top of the ball and the hands underneath the shoulders and on the mat with the elbows straight. The legs are straight and extended from the hips, shoulder-distance apart. Inhale as you draw the belly in and up toward the spine.

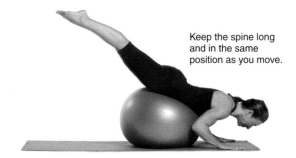

Keep the spine long and in the same position as you move.

2 Exhale as you bend the elbows, bringing the head close to the mat. As the elbows bend, lift the legs toward the ceiling.

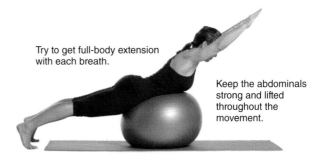

Try to get full-body extension with each breath.

Keep the abdominals strong and lifted throughout the movement.

3 Inhale and lower the legs toward the mat, and as you press the feet into the mat, lift the arms up and over the head, extending the spine. Keep the spine and back from breaking form as you move smoothly through the exercise. Maintain the same spinal curvature and activation throughout the exercise. Repeat from step 2 for 5 to 10 times.

Swimming on the Ball

Press the shoulders down.
Backs of the legs are strong
and contracted.

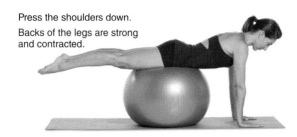

1 Lie on the ball with the hips on top of the ball and
the hands underneath the shoulders and on the mat
with the elbows straight. The legs are straight and
extended from the hips, shoulder-distance apart. Inhale
as you draw the belly in and up toward the spine.

Keep the spine long
and straight.

Move only
the legs.

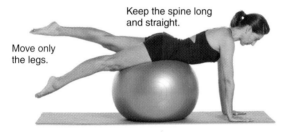

2 Exhale as you flutter kick the legs in small
motions for five counts (approximately 5 seconds).

3 Inhale for five counts as the legs flutter kick.

4 Exhale for five counts as the legs flutter kick.
Repeat steps 3 and 4 for 10 breaths.

Level
▶ Intermediate

Contraindications
▶ Injuries to, chronic conditions
of, or pain in the back, spine,
shoulders, arms, or wrists

Focus
▶ Muscles of the arms, back,
and legs

Benefits
▶ Strengthens the hamstrings
and buttocks
▶ Strengthens the back
muscles
▶ Increases range of motion in
the shoulders
▶ Creates core awareness
▶ Builds coordination

Challenge
To challenge the upper body, move the lower body so that the
feet reach the mat and stay in contact with it as the arms flutter in small, quick motions. You can bend the knees slightly
for more stability or keep them straight and flex the toes under
to grip the floor more securely. Inhale for five counts (approximately 5 seconds) as the arms flutter. Exhale for five counts as
the arms continue to flutter. Repeat for 10 breaths.

Keep the upper body
contracted and lifted.

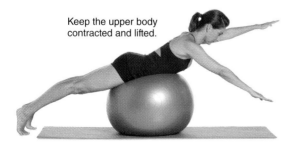

Pike Variations on the Ball

Level

▷ Intermediate to advanced

Contraindications

▷ Injuries to, chronic conditions of, or pain in the back, spine, shoulders, arms, or wrists

Focus

▷ Muscles of the arms, shoulders, back, and legs

Benefits

▷ Strengthens the hamstrings and buttocks
▷ Strengthens the back muscles
▷ Creates core awareness
▷ Builds coordination

BENT-KNEE VARIATION

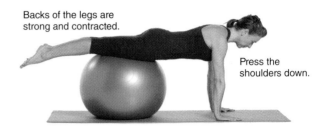

Backs of the legs are strong and contracted.

Press the shoulders down.

1 Lie on the ball with the thighs on top of the ball and the hands underneath the shoulders and on the mat with the elbows straight. The legs are straight and extended from the hips, inner thighs together. Inhale as you draw the belly in and up toward the spine to lengthen the torso.

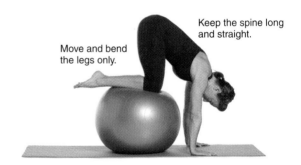

Keep the spine long and straight.

Move and bend the legs only.

2 Exhale as you roll the ball from the thighs to the shins as the knees bend underneath the hips. Inhale as you straighten the legs and return to the start position. Repeat for 8 to 10 repetitions.

STRAIGHT-LEG VARIATION

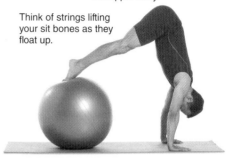

Press into the hands to engage the upper arms and support the upper body.

Think of strings lifting your sit bones as they float up.

1 Start with the ball a little farther down on the thighs than you did for the bent-knee variation. Press into the hands, and take the energy up into the arms to support the shoulders and take the pressure off the wrists. Inhale to prepare, and draw in the belly.

2 Exhale as you bring the ball to the tops of the ankles or the tops of the feet, keeping the legs straight. Make a pike position with the body, like an upside-down V. Inhale as you return the ball to the start position. Repeat for 8 to 10 repetitions.

SINGLE-LEG VARIATION

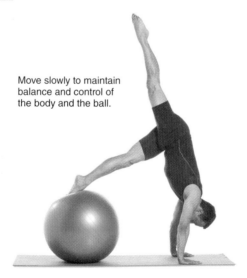

Move slowly to maintain balance and control of the body and the ball.

1 For a challenge to the core, upper body, and legs, lift one leg to the ceiling as you draw the ball underneath you into the pike position.

2 Split the legs as far apart as possible, trying to touch the ceiling with the lifted leg.

Push-Up on the Ball

Level

▶ Intermediate to advanced

Contraindications

▶ Injuries to, chronic conditions of, or pain in the wrists, shoulders, or back

Focus

▶ Muscles of the arms, shoulders, and core

Benefits

▶ Strengthens the arms and shoulders
▶ Teaches core stability

Keep the legs straight as boards.

Lengthen the legs away from the torso.

Engage the upper arms.

Press into the hands and away from the floor.

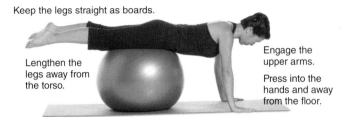

1 Lie over the ball with the hips on top of the ball and the hands on the mat directly below the shoulders, arms straight. Engage the upper arms to take the weight off the wrists.

As the arms bend, keep the body straight and long like a dart.

Shoulders stay away from the ears.

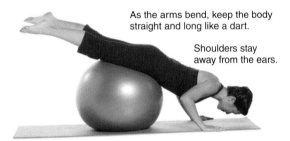

2 Inhale as you bend the elbows, bringing your head as close to the mat as you possibly can without touching it.

Pull the belly in toward the spine.

Move slowly and steadily, balancing the ball under the hips.

Keep the elbows from locking out when they straighten.

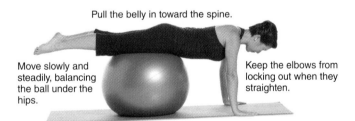

3 Exhale as you straighten the arms, bringing the body back to the start position. Repeat from step 2 for 5 to 10 times.

Challenge

To make the move more challenging, move the body forward off the ball, balancing the thighs on the ball. This is more challenging for the core because you have to lift more of the body with the arms as you push up.

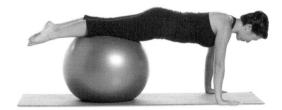

Side-Lying Leg Lift on the Ball

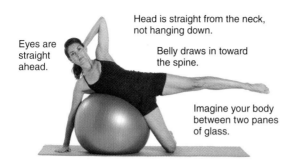

Eyes are straight ahead.

Head is straight from the neck, not hanging down.

Belly draws in toward the spine.

Imagine your body between two panes of glass.

Level
▶ Beginner to intermediate

Contraindications
▶ Injuries to, chronic conditions of, or pain in the arms, wrists, knees, legs, or back

Focus
▶ Muscles of the legs, core, and arms

Benefits
▶ Teaches core stability
▶ Strengthens and stretches the legs
▶ Strengthens the abdominals
▶ Teaches balance and coordination

1 Lie on your right side with the ball under the right rib cage. Bend the right leg, and place that knee on the mat at a 45-degree angle from the hip. Drape your upper body over the ball, and place your hand on the mat on the other side of the ball. The left leg is straight out and hovering above the mat, ready to be worked. The left hand is behind the head, with a bent elbow pointing to the ceiling.

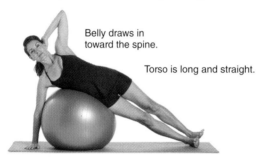

Belly draws in toward the spine.

Torso is long and straight.

Challenge

For more of a challenge, begin in the more challenging position on the stability ball. Lie on your right side with the ball under the right hip. Stretch out both legs, hips and feet stacked on the mat. Drape your upper body from the waist up over the ball, and place your right hand on the mat on the other side of the ball. The left hand is behind the head, with a bent elbow pointing to the ceiling.

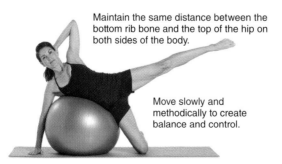

Maintain the same distance between the bottom rib bone and the top of the hip on both sides of the body.

Move slowly and methodically to create balance and control.

2 Inhale as you point the top foot and lift the top leg as high as you can without changing the length of the torso. As you exhale, flex the top foot and lower the leg to the start position. Repeat the lift 8 to 10 times per side.

Side-Lying Leg Circle on the Ball

Level
▶ Beginner to intermediate

Contraindications
▶ Injuries to, chronic conditions of, or pain in the arms, wrists, knees, legs, or back

Focus
▶ Muscles of the leg, core, and arms

Benefits
▶ Teaches core stability
▶ Strengthens and stretches the legs
▶ Strengthens the abdominals
▶ Teaches balance and coordination

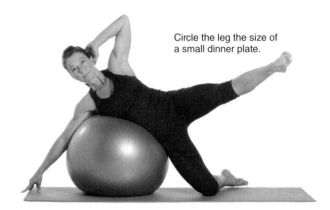

Circle the leg the size of a small dinner plate.

1 Choose your start position on the ball. Inhale as you circle the top leg forward and upward.

2 Exhale as you circle the leg back and down, forming a small circle. Circle the leg for 8 to 10 repetitions, and then reverse the direction and circle for 8 to 10 repetitions.

Side-Lying Front Leg Kick on the Ball

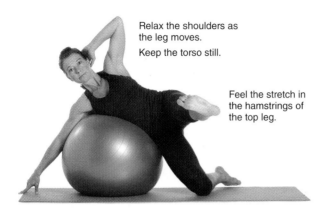

Relax the shoulders as the leg moves.

Keep the torso still.

Feel the stretch in the hamstrings of the top leg.

1 Choose a start side-lying position on the ball. With a double inhale, kick the top leg forward with the foot flexed.

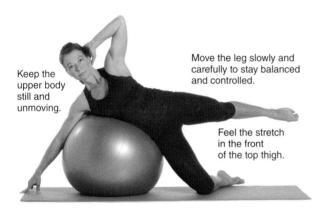

Keep the upper body still and unmoving.

Move the leg slowly and carefully to stay balanced and controlled.

Feel the stretch in the front of the top thigh.

2 Exhale as you kick the top leg back with the foot pointed. Repeat for 8 to 10 times in each direction.

Level
▶ Beginner to intermediate

Contraindications
▶ Injuries to, chronic conditions of, or pain in the arms, wrists, knees, legs, or back

Focus
▶ Muscles of the leg, core, and arms

Benefits
▶ Teaches core stability
▶ Strengthens and stretches the legs
▶ Strengthens the abdominals
▶ Teaches balance and coordination

Side Rollover on the Ball

Level

► Advanced

Contraindications

► Injuries to, chronic conditions of, or pain in the shoulders, back, or spine.

Focus

► Abdominals and muscles of the arms, back, and core

Benefits

► Strengthens the abdominals
► Builds coordination and balance
► Strengthens the arms
► Strengthens the back

Imagine that you are between two sheets of glass.

Abdominals draw in toward the spine.

Eyes are to the front, with the back of the neck long and straight from the spine.

Inner thighs are glued together and strong.

Form a long dartlike position with the body.

1 Lie on your side on the ball with the legs lifted off the mat and the arms on the mat, side by side, shoulder-distance apart. There will be a slight twist to the upper body where the top arm reaches over the body for the mat. Inhale to prepare.

Form a straight, long line with the body, as if you were a board.

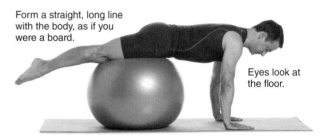

Eyes look at the floor.

2 Exhale as you roll onto the hips and pelvis, facing the floor.

Move slowly and with control.

Keep the body long and straight as you move.

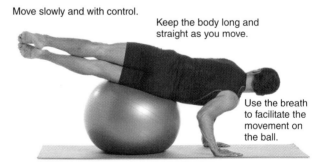

Use the breath to facilitate the movement on the ball.

3 Inhale as you roll to the other side on the other hip. Hands stay on the mat in the same place as the ball moves under the body. Repeat from step 2 for 5 to 10 sets in each direction.

Chapter 9

Pilates Ring Exercises

This chapter features exercises that use the Pilates ring, also called the Magic Circle. The ring is a great accessory to provide extra resistance and to challenge stability and balance in the standard Pilates repertoire. It can also add an element of fun!

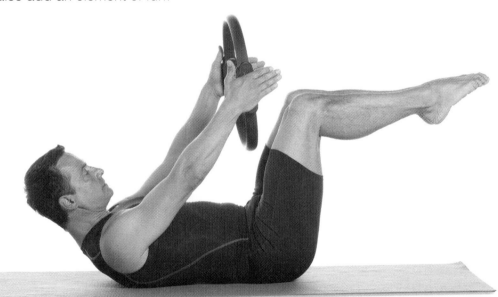

When choosing a ring, look for comfort and weight. Ideally, the Pilates ring should be light to medium weight and have handles (padded is preferred) that you can use from the inside or outside. This type of ring is the most versatile, comfortable, and easiest to use.

Be cautious when using the ring if you have strains or instability in the groin, pubic bone, or sacroiliac joint; ankle, knee, or wrist pain; injuries; or chronic conditions. Since the ring is used mostly between the knees, ankles, or hands, these areas are particularly sensitive to pressure. Avoid using the ring in these areas if you experience pain or injury.

In general the Pilates ring is a very safe accessory, but when exerting extreme pressure on the ring, it can spring away from you or into you. Avoid trying to close the ring. Instead think of applying light to medium pressure to the point of slight exertion on the muscle group being addressed. Working this way also will ensure you are not overworking your stability and posture muscles.

Standing Single-Leg Series: Balance

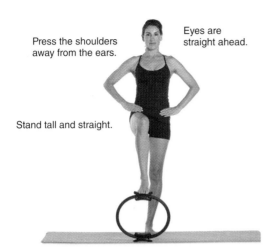

Press the shoulders away from the ears.

Eyes are straight ahead.

Stand tall and straight.

Level
- Beginner

Contraindications
- Injuries to, pain in, or chronic conditions of the ankles, knees, hips, or sacrum

Focus
- Muscles of the legs, buttocks, and core

Benefits
- Strengthens hamstrings
- Teaches balance and coordination
- Builds knee and ankle stability

1 **Stand on one leg with the Pilates ring under the arch of the lifted foot. Hold the hands at the hips or hold the arms straight out from the shoulders with the palms down. If necessary, hold onto a wall to help maintain your balance. Inhale to prepare and balance.**

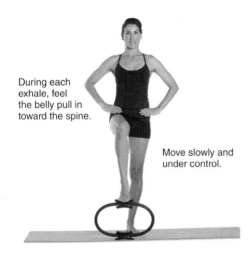

During each exhale, feel the belly pull in toward the spine.

Move slowly and under control.

Variation
An optional standing position is with the arms held out to the sides, palms down.

2 **Exhale as you press the ring down toward the floor. Keep the pressure constant, moving from light to medium resistance with each inhale and exhale.**

3 **Inhale and slightly release the pressure on the ring as you return to the start position under control. Feel grounded on the standing leg to maintain balance and control. Maintain some pressure on the ring at all times. Repeat for 8 to 10 repetitions. Switch sides, and repeat on the other foot for 8 to 10 repetitions. Your balance might feel different on each side.**

Standing Single-Leg Series: Front, Side, and Back

Level

▶ Beginner

Contraindications

▶ Injuries to, pain in, or chronic conditions of the ankles, knees, hips, or sacrum

Focus

▶ Muscles of the legs, buttocks, and core

Benefits

▶ Strengthens inner thighs
▶ Teaches balance and coordination

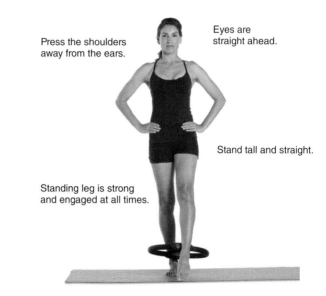

Press the shoulders away from the ears.

Eyes are straight ahead.

Stand tall and straight.

Standing leg is strong and engaged at all times.

1 Stand on one leg with the Pilates ring between your ankles. Begin with the ring in front of the standing leg, with the back of the free ankle holding the ring in front of the standing leg. The hands can be on your hips or at your sides. If necessary, brace yourself against a wall to maintain your balance. Inhale to prepare and balance.

2 Exhale as you press the ring in toward the standing leg. Maintain some pressure on the ring at all times so it doesn't drop to the floor. Use only light to medium pressure on the ring. Feel the belly pull in toward the spine. Repeat in this position for 8 to 10 repetitions.

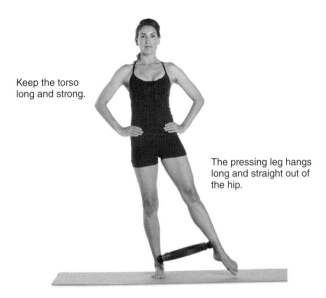

Keep the torso long and strong.

The pressing leg hangs long and straight out of the hip.

3 Inhale as you carefully move the ring to the side of the standing foot. If the ring drops, simply return it to the proper place and continue. If necessary, touch the toes of the free leg to the floor to help your balance.

4 Exhale and press the ring in toward the standing leg. Engage the muscles in the standing leg throughout the exercise, focusing on the inner thigh. Repeat this pulsing action for 8 to 10 repetitions.

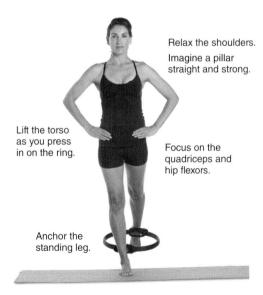

Relax the shoulders.

Imagine a pillar straight and strong.

Lift the torso as you press in on the ring.

Focus on the quadriceps and hip flexors.

Anchor the standing leg.

5 Inhale as you carefully move the ring to the back side of the standing foot.

6 Exhale as you press the ring in toward the standing leg. Repeat in this position for 8 to 10 repetitions. Switch legs, and repeat from step 1 on the other leg. Your balance might feel different on each side. If your standing leg fatigues, switch legs after each repetition to give your standing leg a break.

Standing Arm Series

Level
▶ Beginner

Contraindications
▶ Pain in, injuries to, or chronic conditions of the hands, wrists, elbows, or shoulders

Focus
▶ Muscles of the chest, arms, shoulders, and upper back

Benefits
▶ Strengthens the arms
▶ Strengthens the back
▶ Teaches correct posture for standing tall and straight

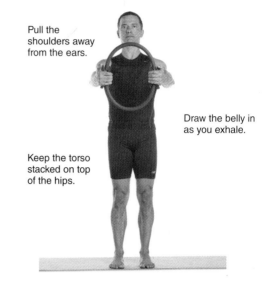

Pull the shoulders away from the ears.

Keep the torso stacked on top of the hips.

Draw the belly in as you exhale.

1 Stand in modified Pilates stance (page 12). Hold the ring in both hands at shoulder height, palms turned in to hold the ring. Apply gentle pressure, enough to feel the chest working and secure the ring between the hands. Inhale to prepare.

2 Exhale as you gently squeeze the ring. Feel the chest muscles engage as you squeeze the ring. Use light to medium pressure on the ring. Inhale as you slowly release. Repeat for 8 to 10 breaths.

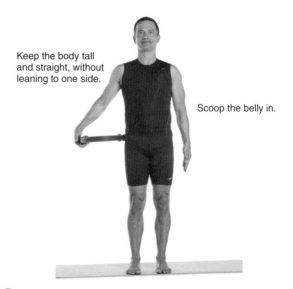

Keep the body tall and straight, without leaning to one side.

Scoop the belly in.

3 Stand in modified Pilates stance. Hold the ring at your hip with one hand. Inhale to prepare.

4 Exhale as you gently squeeze the ring to contract the chest and the latissimus dorsi (the muscles along the sides of your back). Anchor the feet and reach through the top of the head to lengthen the torso. Inhale as you return to the start position. Repeat for 8 to 10 repetitions on one arm, and then switch sides.

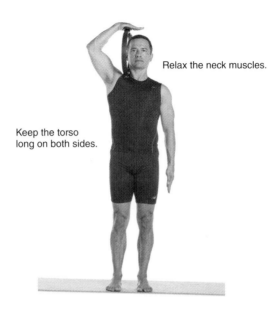

Relax the neck muscles.

Keep the torso long on both sides.

5 Stand in modified Pilates stance. Hold the ring at your shoulder with hand on the same side. Inhale to prepare.

6 Exhale as you gently squeeze the ring down toward the shoulder. Feel the biceps and latissimus dorsi contract to stabilize the torso. Focus on your breath. Repeat for 8 to 10 repetitions on one arm, and then switch to the other side.

Roll-Up With the Ring

Level

▶ Beginner to intermediate

Contraindications

▶ Pain in, injuries to, or chronic conditions of the spine, neck, or back

Focus

▶ Abdominals and muscles of the back and scapulae

Benefits

▶ Strengthens the abdominals
▶ Strengthens the shoulder stabilizers
▶ Increases lower back flexibility
▶ Teaches spinal articulation

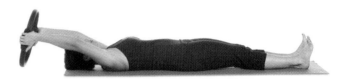

1 Lie down on the mat with the Pilates ring between the hands and the arms, which are extended above the head. If your lower back is particularly tight, choose the supported neutral starting position that is explained in chapter 6 (page 59), as this will aid you in rolling through the tightness in the lower spine.

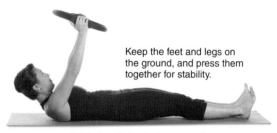

Keep the feet and legs on the ground, and press them together for stability.

Pull in the abdominals to stretch and support the lower spine.

2 Inhale as you lift the arms to the ceiling and bring the chin toward the chest. Roll the head and then the spine off the mat one vertebra at a time. Gently squeeze the ring to help you roll up and off the mat. You can bend your knees, if necessary, to help you roll up.

Pull the shoulders away from the ears as you reach forward.

Keep the lower spine rounded.

Scoop the abdominal wall to support the lower spine.

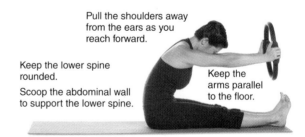

Keep the arms parallel to the floor.

3 Exhale as you continue to roll up and forward until the arms are parallel to the floor and over the legs.

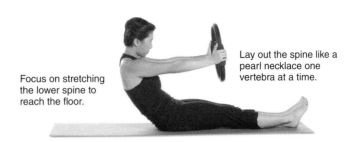

Focus on stretching the lower spine to reach the floor.

Lay out the spine like a pearl necklace one vertebra at a time.

4 Inhale as you begin to roll back, keeping the arms in front of the chest as you roll down. You can bend your knees, if necessary.

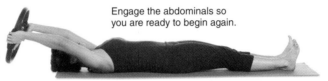

Feel the length of the body as you reach your arms and legs in opposite directions.

Engage the abdominals so you are ready to begin again.

Press the lower back part of the rib cage into the mat.

5 Exhale as you continue to roll down and back until the arms are over the head and the head is on the mat. Repeat steps 2 to 5 for five to eight times.

Rollover With the Ring

Level

▶ Intermediate

Contraindications

▶ Pain in, injuries to, or chronic conditions of the spine, neck, or back

Focus

▶ Abdominals and muscles of the back and scapulae

Benefits

▶ Strengthens the abdominals
▶ Increases lower back flexibility
▶ Teaches spinal articulation

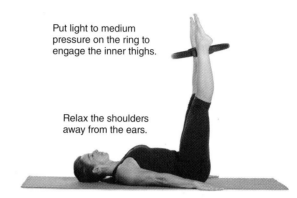

Put light to medium pressure on the ring to engage the inner thighs.

Relax the shoulders away from the ears.

1 Lie on the mat with the Pilates ring between the ankles, the legs extended straight above your hips and the toes pointed toward the ceiling. The arms are beside the body with the palms turned down. Inhale and pull the abdominals in. Slightly press the palms into the mat to prepare the body. You can bend your knees slightly, if necessary.

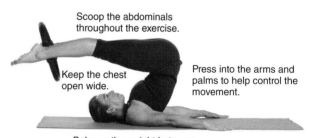

Scoop the abdominals throughout the exercise.

Keep the chest open wide.

Press into the arms and palms to help control the movement.

Balance the weight between your shoulder blades.

2 Exhale as you press into the hands and roll the hips over the spine until the legs are parallel to the floor above the head and the ring is reaching toward the wall behind you.

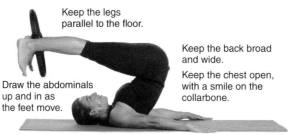

Keep the legs parallel to the floor.

Keep the back broad and wide.

Keep the chest open, with a smile on the collarbone.

Draw the abdominals up and in as the feet move.

Relax the neck area.

3 Inhale as you flex the feet and press into the ring a bit more.

4 Exhale as you roll back down the spine until the legs are just above the hips. Move slowly on the return to lengthen the spine. Use your abdominals to control the descent of the spine.

5 Inhale and point the toes to the ceiling. Feel the sit bones lengthen toward the floor as the feet reach for the ceiling. Repeat for four to six repetitions.

Single-Leg Stretch With the Ring

Level

► Beginner to intermediate

Contraindications

► Pain in, injuries to, or chronic conditions of the spine, neck, back, arms, or shoulders

Focus

► Abdominals and muscles of the back and arms

Benefits

► Strengthens the abdominals
► Increases upper back flexibility
► Teaches core control
► Teaches breath and movement coordination
► Builds arm and shoulder stability and strength

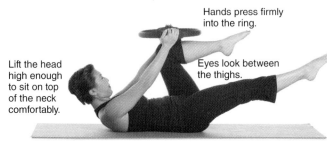

Hands press firmly into the ring.

Lift the head high enough to sit on top of the neck comfortably.

Eyes look between the thighs.

Relax the shoulders and the neck.

Press the belly toward the spine.

1 Lie on your back on the mat with one knee above the hip and the other leg stretched out at a 45-degree angle above the floor. Lift your head, neck, and shoulders off the mat. The arms are outstretched, with the Pilates ring between the hands and above the shins. Inhale and prepare.

2 Exhale as you switch the legs twice, keeping the arms in position with the ring just above the shins. Feel the inner thighs and knees touch lightly as they pass each other. Focus on your breath to coordinate the movement. Continue to switch legs for 5 to 10 repetitions, alternating two leg movements on each inhale and two on each exhale.

Double-Leg Stretch With the Ring

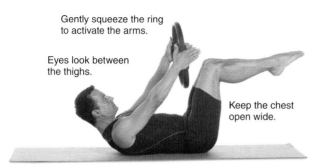

Gently squeeze the ring to activate the arms.

Eyes look between the thighs.

Keep the chest open wide.

1 Lie on your back with the knees above the hips in tabletop position. Hold the Pilates ring in your hands above the shins with the head lifted.

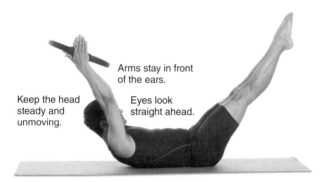

Arms stay in front of the ears.

Keep the head steady and unmoving.

Eyes look straight ahead.

2 Inhale as you stretch the arms up by the ears and the legs straight out to a 45-degree position.

3 Exhale as you return to tabletop position. Use the exhale to deepen the scoop in the abdominals. Move slowly and under control. Repeat for four to eight repetitions.

Level
▶ Beginner to intermediate

Contraindications
▶ Injuries to, pain in, or chronic conditions of the spine, neck, back, or shoulders

Focus
▶ Abdominals and muscles of the back, arms, and shoulders

Benefits
▶ Strengthens the abdominals
▶ Increases upper back flexibility
▶ Teaches core control
▶ Builds coordination of arm and leg movement with breath

Double Straight-Leg Stretch With the Ring

Level
▶ Intermediate

Contraindications
▶ Injuries to, pain in, or chronic conditions of the spine, neck, back, or shoulders

Focus
▶ Abdominals and muscles of the back, arms, and shoulders

Benefits
▶ Strengthens the abdominals
▶ Increases upper back flexibility
▶ Teaches core control
▶ Builds coordination of arm and leg movement with breath

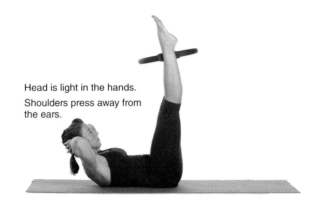

Head is light in the hands.
Shoulders press away from the ears.

1 Lie down on your back with the hands supporting the head, elbows wide and head lifted. Legs are straight and pointed to the ceiling, with the ring between the ankles.

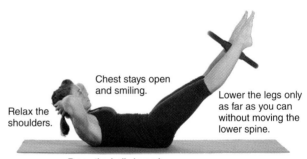

Chest stays open and smiling.

Relax the shoulders.

Lower the legs only as far as you can without moving the lower spine.

Press the belly in and down to support the back.

2 Inhale as you extend the legs to a 45-degree position.

3 Exhale as you return to the start position with the legs above the hips. Use your breath to deepen the abdominal contraction. Move slowly to control each movement. Repeat for four to eight repetitions.

Crisscross With the Ring

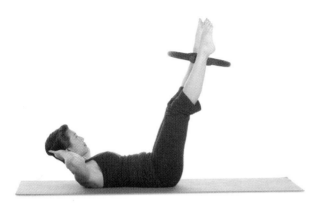

1 Lie on your back with the hands behind the head to support the neck and the legs stretched out straight above the hips, with the Pilates ring between the ankles. Bend your knees slightly if your hamstring flexibility is limited. Inhale and prepare.

Level
▶ Intermediate

Contraindications
▶ Injuries to, pain in, or chronic conditions of the spine, neck, back, or shoulders

Focus
▶ Abdominals and muscles of the back, arms, and shoulders

Benefits
▶ Strengthens the abdominals
▶ Increases upper back flexibility
▶ Teaches core control
▶ Builds coordination of arm and leg movement with breath

Keep the elbows wide.

The movement comes from the torso and waist, deep in the obliques.

Move slowly to maintain control of the Pilates ring.

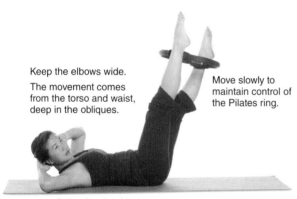

Relax the shoulders.

2 Exhale as you rotate one leg toward the chest and the opposite side of the upper body in toward that leg. Repeat to the other direction while still exhaling. If necessary, readjust the ring between the ankles.

3 Inhale to alternate the legs and upper body twice. Maintain light to medium pressure on the ring for control. Relax the shoulders and keep them pressed down away from the ears. Repeat for four to eight breaths.

Teaser Variations With the Ring

Level

▶ Intermediate to advanced

Contraindications

▶ Pain in, injuries to, or chronic conditions of the spine, neck, or back

Focus

▶ Abdominals and legs

Benefits

▶ Strengthens the abdominals and hip flexors

▶ Develops coordination and balance

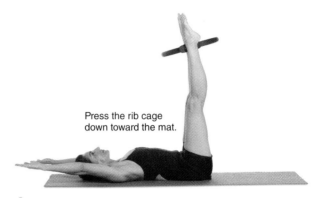

Press the rib cage down toward the mat.

1 Lie on your back with the legs straight above the hips and the Pilates ring between the ankles. The arms are straight and reaching over the head. (They might be just above the mat if the shoulder area is tight.)

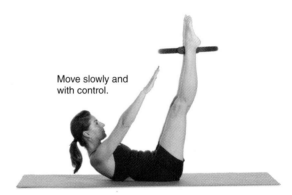

Move slowly and with control.

2 Inhale as you lift the arms to the ceiling and begin to peel the head, neck, and shoulders off the mat. The legs will begin to lower toward 45 degrees.

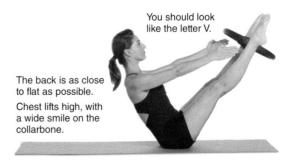

You should look like the letter V.

The back is as close to flat as possible.

Chest lifts high, with a wide smile on the collarbone.

3 Exhale as you continue to roll up and the legs extend at a 45-degree angle above the mat. Arms reach up toward the ankles.

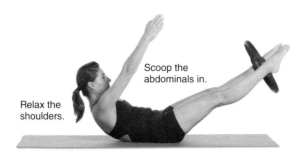

Relax the
shoulders.

Scoop the
abdominals in.

4 Inhale as you begin to roll down the spine toward the mat. Keep the arms stretching forward. The legs will begin to lower toward the mat.

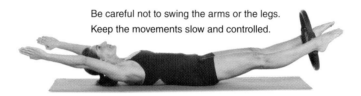

Be careful not to swing the arms or the legs.
Keep the movements slow and controlled.

5 Exhale as you continue to roll down, bringing the arms above the head to the start position and the legs to a position just off the mat. Repeat for three to five repetitions.

Advanced Variation

From step 3, inhale and grab the ankles. Exhale and roll back like Open Leg Rocker (chapter 7, page 99). Inhale to take a sip of air at the bottom. Exhale and roll back up to the teaser position. Repeat for three to five repetitions, and then release the ankles and continue from step 4 to the finish.

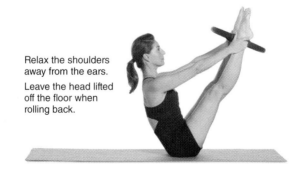

Relax the shoulders away from the ears.

Leave the head lifted off the floor when rolling back.

Swan With the Ring

Level

▶ Intermediate

Contraindications

▶ Pain in, injuries to, or chronic conditions of the lower back, shoulders, elbows, or wrists

Focus

▶ Hamstrings and muscles of the upper back and shoulders

Benefits

▶ Strengthens the hamstrings, back extensors, and buttocks
▶ Stretches the abdominals
▶ Improves shoulder stability
▶ Improves back extension

Gently squeeze the buttocks to press the pubic bone into the mat and lengthen the lower spine.

Draw the shoulder blades away from the ears and down the back.

Pull the belly button in toward the spine.

1 Lie on your abdomen with your forehead on the mat, hands along the outside edges of the Pilates ring, palms turned in. Inner thighs are sit-bone-distance apart, with both legs contracted and the belly drawn in away from the mat. Inhale to prepare.

Lift the sternum to open the chest.

Eyes look straight ahead to keep the neck in alignment with the torso.

Gently contract the buttocks to protect and lengthen the lower spine.

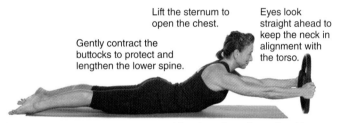

Lift only as far as is comfortable for the lower back.

2 Exhale as you press the hands into the ring and lift your upper body.

3 Inhale to return to the start position. Feel the body lengthen with the breath. Repeat for four to six repetitions.

Single-Leg Press

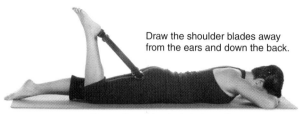

Draw the shoulder blades away from the ears and down the back.

Scoop the abdominals in by pulling the belly button in toward the spine.

1 **Lie on your abdomen. Place the Pilates ring against the ankle or heel and between the fold of the buttocks and the leg on one side of the body. Rest the forehead on the backs of the hands, which are folded on the mat, palms down. Inhale to prepare.**

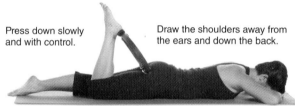

Press down slowly and with control.

Draw the shoulders away from the ears and down the back.

Pull the belly in toward the spine.

2 **Exhale as you press the ankle on the ring toward the floor. Keep energy through the extended leg along the mat, lengthening it away from the torso.**

3 **Inhale as you return to the start position. Release the tension slowly to remain in control of the ring. Repeat for 8 to 10 repetitions. Repeat the same exercise on the other side.**

Level
▶ Intermediate

Contraindications
▶ Pain in, injuries to, or chronic conditions of the lower back, knees, ankles, or hips

Focus
▶ Hamstrings and buttocks

Benefits
▶ Strengthens the hamstrings
▶ Strengthens the buttocks

Side-Lying Top Leg Press Down With the Ring

Level
► Beginner to intermediate

Contraindications
► Sensitivity in the outer hip area (greater trochanter)
► Pain in, injuries to, or chronic conditions of the hips, legs, knees, ankles, neck, shoulders, elbows, or wrists

Focus
► Inner thighs

Benefits
► Promotes control and stability in the hips, pelvis, and torso
► Strengthens the hip, buttock, and inner thigh muscles

Feel the waist pull up from the mat and lengthen away from your ribs.

Flex the feet as if you were standing on them.

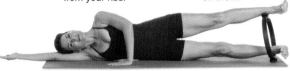

1 Lie on your side with your torso lined up straight along the back edge of the mat. Flex the hips so that the legs are slightly in front of your body. Place the bottom leg inside the Pilates ring and the top leg on top of the Pilates ring. Flex the feet toward the body. Lay your head over the right arm, with the palm turned up or down. The right elbow can be bent to cradle your head, if necessary. Bend the top elbow, and place the hand in front of the body for support. Inhale to prepare.

2 Exhale as you press down with the top leg. Keep the torso long and straight as you move and relax the shoulders. Repeat 8 to 10 times on each leg.

Side-Lying Top Leg Press Up With the Ring

Feel the top leg reach away
from the hip as it lifts.

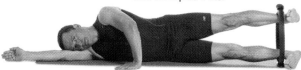

Contract the bottom leg to
help balance the body.

1 In the side-lying position, place the top leg on the inside of the Pilates ring, touching the inside top of the ring at the ankle. Inhale to prepare.

2 Exhale to press the top leg up toward the ceiling. Inhale to return the ring to its original shape. When releasing pressure on the ring, always move slowly and precisely. Try to resist the release of tension when you let up on the pressure on the ring. Repeat 8 to 10 times. You can go on to the next side-lying exercise on this side or repeat this exercise on the other side.

Level

▶ Beginner to intermediate

Contraindications

▶ Sensitivity in the outer hip area (greater trochanter)
▶ Pain in, injuries to, or chronic conditions of the hips, legs, knees, ankles, neck, shoulders, elbows, or wrists

Focus

▶ Outer thighs and external rotators

Benefits

▶ Promotes control and stability in the hips, pelvis, and torso
▶ Strengthens the hip, buttock, and inner thigh muscles

Side-Lying Leg Circle With the Ring

Level

▶ Beginner to intermediate

Contraindications

▶ Sensitivity in the outer hip area (greater trochanter)
▶ Pain in, injuries to, or chronic conditions of the hips, legs, knees, ankles, neck, shoulders, elbows, or wrists

Focus

▶ Inner and outer thighs and external rotators

Benefits

▶ Promotes control and stability in the hips, pelvis, and torso
▶ Strengthens the hip, buttock, and inner thigh muscles

Steady and relax the upper body.

Maintain the length of the torso as you circle the leg.

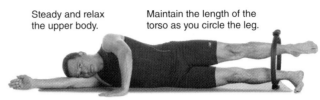

Keep both legs strong and activated.

1 In the side-lying position, place the top leg inside the Pilates ring toward the top, front edge. Inhale as you begin a small circle of the leg inside the ring toward the front and down.

2 Exhale as you continue to circle back and up to the start position. Repeat this forward circle for 8 to 10 repetitions, and then repeat in the other direction. You can go on to the next side-lying exercise on this side or repeat this exercise on the other side.

Side-Lying Bicycle With the Ring

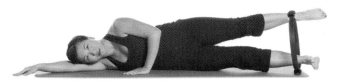

1 In the side-lying position, place the top leg at hip height behind the bottom leg and the Pilates ring.

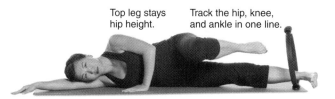

Top leg stays hip height.

Track the hip, knee, and ankle in one line.

2 Inhale as you bend the top knee, keeping the knee hip height.

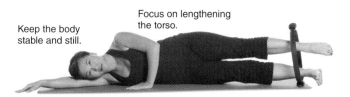

Keep the body stable and still.

Focus on lengthening the torso.

3 Exhale and straighten the top leg through the ring, keeping the toes pointed.

4 Inhale as you bend the top knee, bringing the toes from the middle of the ring to in front of the hip. Exhale and straighten the leg, returning it to the front of the ring. Repeat, bending the knee and changing the foot placement from front to center to back, for three to five cycles. You can go on to the next side-lying exercise on this side or repeat this exercise on the other side.

Level
▶ Beginner to intermediate

Contraindications
▶ Sensitivity in the outer hip area (greater trochanter)
▶ Pain in, injuries to, or chronic conditions of the hips, legs, knees, ankles, neck, shoulders, elbows, or wrists

Focus
▶ Inner and outer thighs, external rotators, hamstrings, hip flexors, and buttocks

Benefits
▶ Promotes control and stability in the hips, pelvis, and torso
▶ Strengthens the hip, buttock, and inner thigh muscles

Leg Tap With the Ring

Level

▶ Beginner to intermediate

Contraindications

▶ Sensitivity in the outer hip area (greater trochanter)
▶ Pain in, injuries to, or chronic conditions of the hips, legs, knees, ankles, neck, shoulders, elbows, or wrists

Focus

▶ Inner and outer thighs and external rotators

Benefits

▶ Promotes control and stability in the hips, pelvis, and torso
▶ Strengthens the hip, buttock, and inner thigh muscles

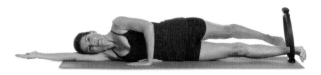

1 In the side-lying position, place the top leg at hip height behind the bottom leg and the Pilates ring.

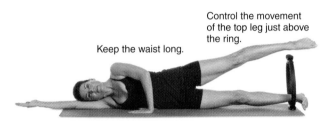

Control the movement of the top leg just above the ring.

Keep the waist long.

2 Inhale as you circle the leg above the ring.

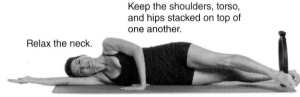

Keep the shoulders, torso, and hips stacked on top of one another.

Relax the neck.

Bottom leg stays long.

3 Continue to inhale, and make a half circle above the ring with the top leg. Bring it over to the front of the ring.

4 Exhale as you make a half circle to the back of the ring. Repeat this half circle for four to eight breaths or repetitions.

Chapter 10

Band Exercises

This chapter features exercises that use the elastic band. Traditionally this prop is used as a tool in physical therapy for rehabilitation and for patients to use at home with therapy exercises. Here, we use the band either to provide support to make an exercise easier or, in some cases, as a tool to provide resistance to make some exercises more challenging. The band is very small, light, and easy to use; you can take it with you almost anywhere; and it can be used in a small space.

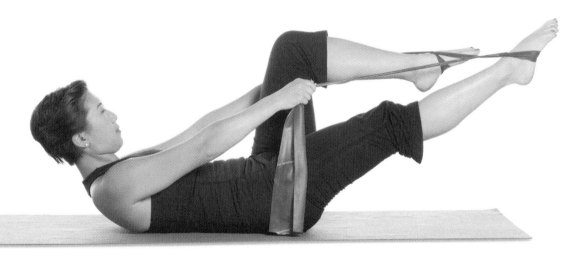

Bands come in different colors, each color representing a different level of resistance. For the most part, you want to choose a band with low- to medium-level resistance. Remember, the goal is not to strain but to strengthen with length. The band should be at least 6 feet (1.8 m) long so that you will not strain or break it during exercise. Some bands come with handles, or you can purchase handles separately, to make gripping the band easier.

There are some simple rules for using the band. If you notice any tear in the band, do not use it. It may break during exercise and snap into you or someone or something around you. Hold the band gently. Refrain from wrapping the band around the hand or foot several times as this may cut off your circulation as you pull the band during exercise.

There are several ways to use the band correctly. Figures 10.1 through 10.5 show the most common ways.

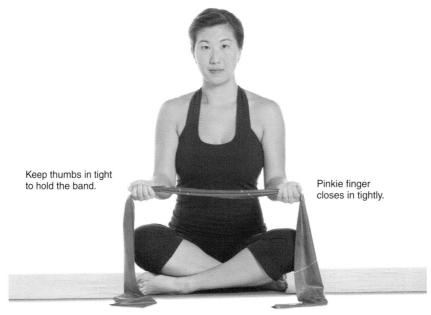

Keep thumbs in tight to hold the band.

Pinkie finger closes in tightly.

Figure 10.1   With the palms turned up, place the band across the hands, allowing the band to come over the palms and between the thumbs. Close the thumbs to the sides of the hands to secure the band, and then curl the fingers toward the palms, pulling in tight, especially with the pinkie finger.

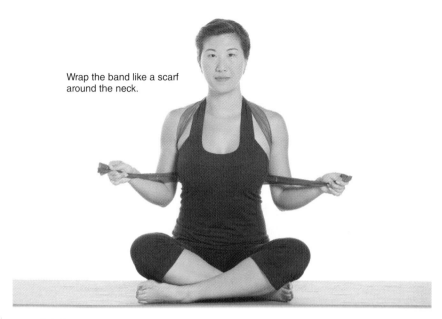

Wrap the band like a scarf around the neck.

Figure 10.2 Wrap the band around the neck, cross it behind you, and pull the ends underneath the arms and around the sides of the body.

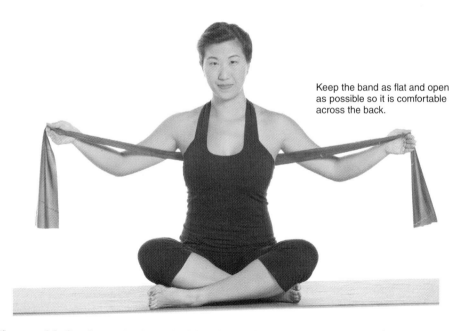

Keep the band as flat and open as possible so it is comfortable across the back.

Figure 10.3 Cross the band behind the body, and then take hold of one end in each hand in front of the body.

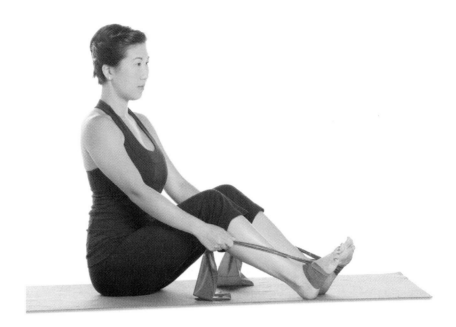

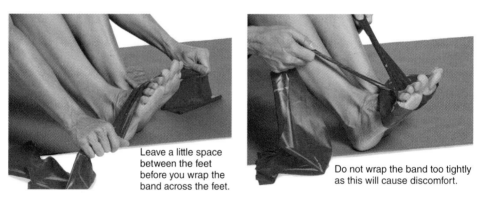

Leave a little space between the feet before you wrap the band across the feet.

Do not wrap the band too tightly as this will cause discomfort.

Figure 10.4 Place the band over the tops of the feet, with the ends on the outside edge of the feet. Wrap the ends under the balls of the feet, and then pull the band between the feet and take hold of one end in each hand.

Typically bands are packaged with a powdered finish. If you have skin sensitivity or conditions, exercise caution when using the band. You may want to test the band on your skin first to be sure it will not cause a reaction.

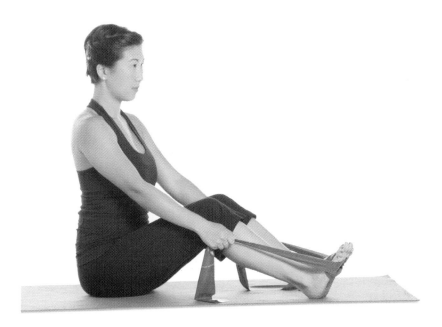

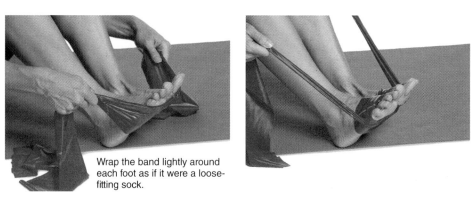

Wrap the band lightly around each foot as if it were a loose-fitting sock.

Figure 10.5 Place the band underneath the balls of the feet, with the ends coming toward the torso from the outside edge of each foot. Wrap the band around each foot, and bring the ends between the feet and around the outside of each foot.

Be sure not to break form at the wrists; keep the wrists in a straight position. If you break form at the wrists or smaller joints when pulling on the band, the pressure may cause pain and possibly injury to that part of the body.

Standing Stretches With the Band

Level

▶ Beginner

Contraindications

▶ Injuries to, pain in, or chronic conditions of the wrists, elbows, knees, hips, or back

Focus

▶ Muscles of the arms and upper body

Benefits

▶ Increases flexibility in the upper back and chest
▶ Increases lateral flexion (side of the body)
▶ Teaches balance and coordination

SIDE STRETCH

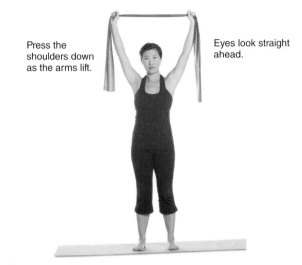

Press the shoulders down as the arms lift.

Eyes look straight ahead.

1 Stand in modified Pilates stance (page 12). Hold one end of the band in each hand, and lift the arms above the head.

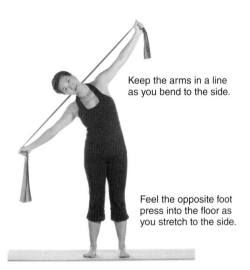

Keep the arms in a line as you bend to the side.

Feel the opposite foot press into the floor as you stretch to the side.

2 Inhale as you bend to one side. Pull the band down with the arm on the same side you are stretching toward.

3 Exhale as you return to the start position. Inhale and bend to the other side. Reach up and over the feet as you move from side to side. Feel as if your body is between two panes of glass. Repeat for four to six sets, alternating sides.

UPPER BACK STRETCH

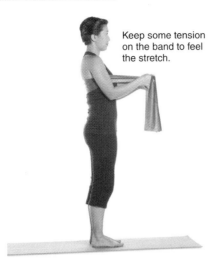

Keep some tension on the band to feel the stretch.

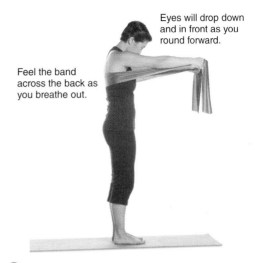

Eyes will drop down and in front as you round forward.

Feel the band across the back as you breathe out.

1 Hold one end of the band in each hand, and wrap the band across the upper back and under the arms. Bend the elbows and inhale deeply.

2 Exhale as you straighten both arms. Reach forward as you round the upper back only.

3 Inhale as you return to the start position by bending the elbows and straightening the upper back. Eyes look straight ahead. Repeat for four to six repetitions.

CHEST STRETCH

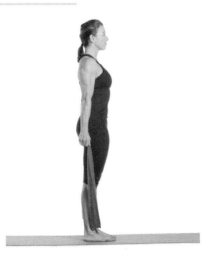

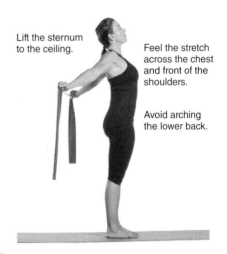

Lift the sternum to the ceiling.

Feel the stretch across the chest and front of the shoulders.

Avoid arching the lower back.

1 Hold an end of the band in each hand, with the arms hanging straight down and the band hanging behind the body. To increase the stretch, hold the hands closer together with more tension in the band.

2 Inhale as you lift the chest and lift the arms behind you. Exhale as you return to the start position. Repeat for four to eight repetitions.

Side Arm Lunge Series

Level
▶ Beginner to advanced

Contraindications
▶ Injuries to, pain in, or chronic conditions of the wrists, elbows, knees, hips, or back

Focus
▶ Muscles of the arms, legs, buttocks, and core

Benefits
▶ Strengthens arms
▶ Strengthens legs
▶ Teaches balance and coordination

BEGINNER

1 **Stand facing forward with the feet parallel and under the sit bones. Place one end of the band under your left foot, keeping a small portion hanging to the side of that foot. Hold the other end of the band in the right hand. Hold the right elbow under the shoulder and the right hand across the waist in the start position. Inhale to prepare.**

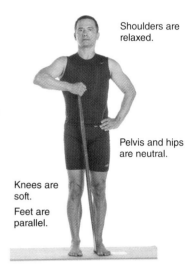

Shoulders are relaxed.

Pelvis and hips are neutral.

Knees are soft.

Feet are parallel.

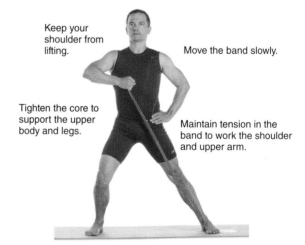

Keep your shoulder from lifting.

Move the band slowly.

Tighten the core to support the upper body and legs.

Maintain tension in the band to work the shoulder and upper arm.

2 Exhale as you step the right foot out in a lunge to the side and slightly to the front. As you lunge, pull the band to the right side of the body, keeping the elbow bent, like a row. The nonworking hand is at the hip with the elbow pointed out. Eyes look straight ahead.

3 Inhale as you return the arm back to the start position in front of the body and the right foot back to parallel under the hip. Resist the return of the band to the start position. Keep the upper body tall and straight and press the shoulders away from the ears. Repeat for 8 to 10 repetitions.

INTERMEDIATE

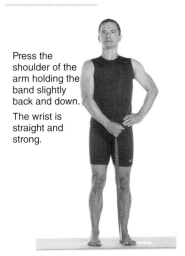

Press the shoulder of the arm holding the band slightly back and down.

The wrist is straight and strong.

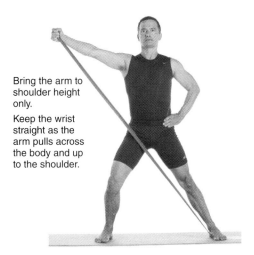

Bring the arm to shoulder height only.

Keep the wrist straight as the arm pulls across the body and up to the shoulder.

1 The legs start in the same position as for the beginner version. With this variation, the moving arm will remain straight. Inhale to prepare.

2 Exhale as you lunge to the side and pull the arm straight across the body and out to the side in a lateral raise.

3 Inhale as you slowly return the arm to the start position. Press the shoulders down and away from the ears. Engage the muscles of the moving arm and keep it strong. Repeat for 8 to 10 repetitions.

ADVANCED

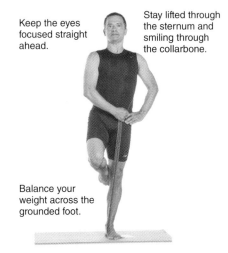

Keep the eyes focused straight ahead.

Stay lifted through the sternum and smiling through the collarbone.

Balance your weight across the grounded foot.

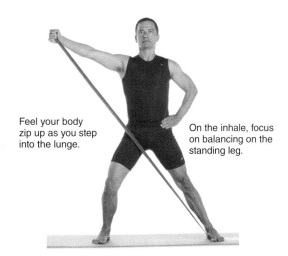

Feel your body zip up as you step into the lunge.

On the inhale, focus on balancing on the standing leg.

1 From the same start position as for the beginner version, inhale and lift the right knee to hip height.

2 Step out into a lunge with the right foot, and perform the arm movement from either the beginner or intermediate version. Repeat for 8 to 10 repetitions on each side.

Double-Arm Lunge Series

Level

▸ Beginner to intermediate

Contraindications

▸ Injuries to, pain in, or chronic conditions of the wrists, elbows, knees, hips, or back

Focus

▸ Muscles of the arms, legs, buttocks, and core

Benefits

▸ Strengthens arms
▸ Strengthens legs
▸ Teaches balance and coordination

DOUBLE-ARM BICEPS LUNGE

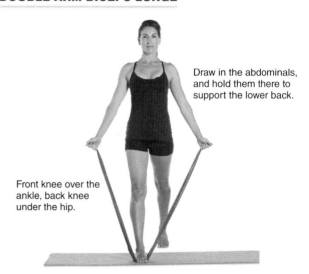

Draw in the abdominals, and hold them there to support the lower back.

Front knee over the ankle, back knee under the hip.

1 Place the band across the floor in front of you. Step in the middle of the band, with one foot placed firmly across the center. Take an end of the band in each hand, and lunge back with the free leg. Bend the front leg slightly so the knee is directly over the ankle, and bend the back knee so it is under the hip. The arms hang straight down from the shoulders. Inhale to prepare.

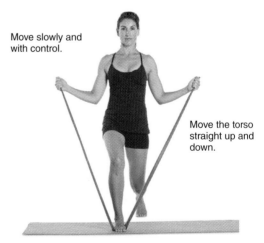

Move slowly and with control.

Move the torso straight up and down.

2 Exhale as you pull the ends of the band toward the ceiling, performing a biceps curl with each arm as you drop deeper into the knee bend. You can adjust the tension of the band by holding it closer to or farther away from the ends.

3 Inhale as you return the band and the legs to the start position. Resist the band on the return. Repeat for 8 to 10 repetitions.

DOUBLE-ARM TRICEPS LUNGE

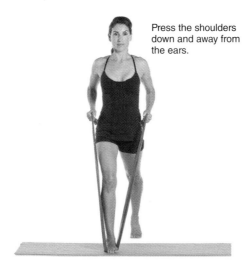

Press the shoulders down and away from the ears.

4 From the start position of Double Arm Biceps Lunge, inhale as you bend both arms at the elbows and lift the elbows toward the ceiling behind you. To make the exercise more or less difficult, adjust the tension on the band by moving your hands up or down on the band.

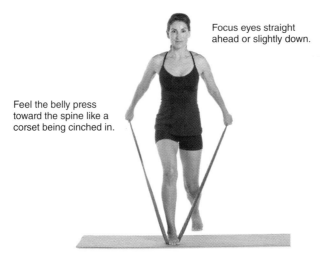

Focus eyes straight ahead or slightly down.

Feel the belly press toward the spine like a corset being cinched in.

5 Exhale as you straighten both arms behind the body in a triceps extension and sink deeper into the knee bend.

6 Inhale as you return the arms to the start position. Repeat for 8 to 10 repetitions.

Spine Twist With the Band

Level
▶ Beginner

Contraindications
▶ Injuries to, pain in, or chronic conditions of the wrists, elbows, or shoulders

Focus
▶ Muscles of the arms, core, and upper body

Benefits
▶ Strengthens the oblique abdominals
▶ Strengthens the arms
▶ Builds coordination and control

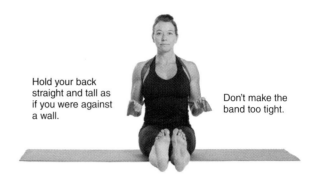

Hold your back straight and tall as if you were against a wall.

Don't make the band too tight.

1 Wrap the band in the harness hold (figure 10.2, page 163). Hold one end of the band in each hand. Make sure the band is loose enough that you can lengthen the arms away from the torso. Arms are bent with the wrists held out to the sides at a 90-degree angle, palms turned up. Inhale to prepare the body.

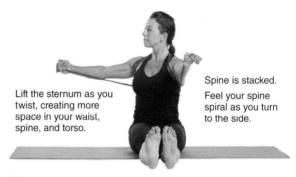

Lift the sternum as you twist, creating more space in your waist, spine, and torso.

Spine is stacked.

Feel your spine spiral as you turn to the side.

2 Exhale as you twist the body to one side and straighten your arms to the sides, pulling the band away from the torso. Keep the spine stacked with the head over the shoulders, the shoulders over the rib cage, and the rib cage over the hips.

3 Inhale as you return to the start position. Bend the elbows back toward the torso.

4 Exhale as you twist to the other side and straighten the arms to the sides. Repeat for four to six sets, alternating sides.

Single-Leg Stretch With the Band

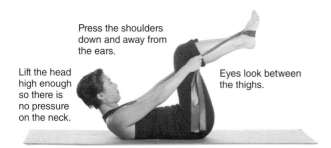

Press the shoulders down and away from the ears.

Lift the head high enough so there is no pressure on the neck.

Eyes look between the thighs.

Level

▶ Beginner to intermediate

Contraindications

▶ Injuries to, pain in, or chronic conditions of the wrists, elbows, knees, hips, or back

Focus

▶ Muscles of the arms, legs, core, and upper body

Benefits

▶ Strengthens the abdominals and arms
▶ Tones the legs
▶ Builds coordination and control

1 Lie on your back. Choose the supine position that best meets your needs according to the guidelines discussed in chapter 6 (pages 58-59). Wrap the band around your feet, with the ends on the inside of the feet. Hold an end of the band in each hand, with the arms reaching up toward either side of the knees. Bring the knees above the hips in tabletop position. Lift the head and upper body off the ground. Inhale to prepare.

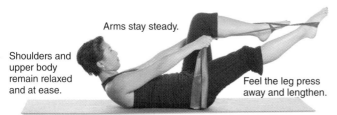

Arms stay steady.

Shoulders and upper body remain relaxed and at ease.

Feel the leg press away and lengthen.

Press the belly in and down toward the mat.

2 Exhale as you extend one leg out straight to a 45-degree position above the floor as the other leg stays in tabletop position. Continue to exhale as you switch legs.

3 Inhale as you switch the legs twice again. Repeat for five to eight sets.

Single Straight-Leg Stretch With the Band

Level

▶ Beginner to intermediate

Contraindications

▶ Injuries to, pain in, or chronic conditions of the wrists, elbows, knees, hips, or back

Focus

▶ Muscles of the arms, legs, core, and upper body

Benefits

▶ Strengthens the abdominals and arms

▶ Tones the legs

▶ Builds coordination and control

▶ Builds leg flexibility

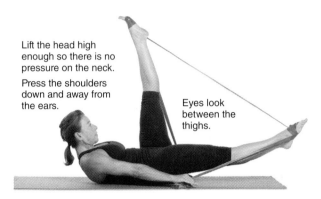

Lift the head high enough so there is no pressure on the neck.

Press the shoulders down and away from the ears.

Eyes look between the thighs.

1 Lie on your back. Choose the supine position that best meets your needs according to the guidelines discussed in chapter 6 (pages 58-59). Wrap the band around your feet, with the ends on the outside of the feet. Keep the band lax between the feet in anticipation of scissoring the legs. The legs are straight, with one leg angled about 45 degrees from the mat and the other leg just above the hip. Hold an end of the band in each hand, with the arms straight out to the sides and just above the mat. Lift the head and upper body off the mat. Inhale to prepare.

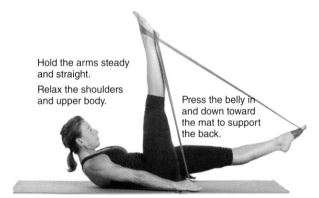

Hold the arms steady and straight.

Relax the shoulders and upper body.

Press the belly in and down toward the mat to support the back.

2 Exhale as you scissor the legs (lower one leg and lift the other) twice, keeping the legs straight. As you scissor the legs, keep reaching the arms out long just above the mat, creating tension in the band to increase arm strength.

3 Inhale as you switch the legs two times again. Repeat for five to eight sets.

Double-Leg Stretch With the Band

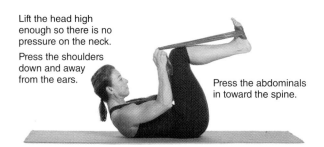

Lift the head high enough so there is no pressure on the neck.

Press the shoulders down and away from the ears.

Press the abdominals in toward the spine.

Level
- ▸ Beginner to intermediate

Contraindications
- ▸ Injuries to, pain in, or chronic conditions of the wrists, elbows, knees, hips, or back

Focus
- ▸ Muscles of the arms, legs, core, and upper body

Benefits
- ▸ Strengthens the abdominals and arms
- ▸ Tones the legs
- ▸ Builds coordination and control

1 Lie on your back. Choose the supine position that best meets your needs according to the guidelines discussed in chapter 6 (pages 58-59). Wrap the band around your feet, with the ends on the outside of the feet. Hold an end of the band in each hand, elbows bent and upper arms hovering just above the mat. Cinch the band so there is slight tension but you can create more as you pull with the arms. Bend the legs and lift them to just above the hips in tabletop position. Lift the head and upper body off the mat.

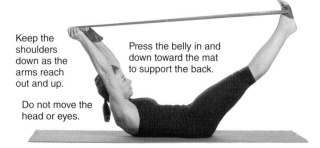

Keep the shoulders down as the arms reach out and up.

Do not move the head or eyes.

Press the belly in and down toward the mat to support the back.

2 Inhale as you extend the legs at a 45-degree angle above the mat. Reach the arms straight above the head and toward the ears.

3 Exhale forcefully as you return to the start position. The forceful exhale will help you engage the abdominals. Repeat for five to eight sets.

Diamond Leg Press

Level

▷ Intermediate

Contraindications

▷ Injuries to, pain in, or chronic conditions of the wrists, elbows, knees, hips, or back

Focus

▷ Muscles of the arms, legs, core, and upper body

Benefits

▷ Strengthens the abdominals
▷ Tones the legs
▷ Strengthens the arms
▷ Builds coordination and control

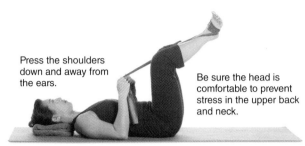

Press the shoulders down and away from the ears.

Be sure the head is comfortable to prevent stress in the upper back and neck.

Anchor the upper arms to the mat.

1 Lie on your back. Choose the supine position that best meets your needs according to the guidelines discussed in chapter 6 (pages 58-59). Wrap the band across the feet with the ends outside the feet. Hold an end of the band in each hand, elbows bent and upper arms on the mat. Cinch the band so there is slight tension but you can create more as you pull with the arms. Bend the legs with the knees out to the sides and just above the hips in turned-out tabletop position. Inhale to prepare.

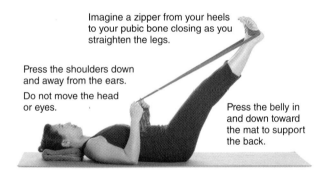

Imagine a zipper from your heels to your pubic bone closing as you straighten the legs.

Press the shoulders down and away from the ears.

Do not move the head or eyes.

Press the belly in and down toward the mat to support the back.

2 Exhale as you straighten and extend the legs at a 45-degree angle above the mat. Bring the inner thighs together, keeping the toes turned out.

3 Inhale as you return to the start position. Repeat for five to eight repetitions.

Rollover With the Band

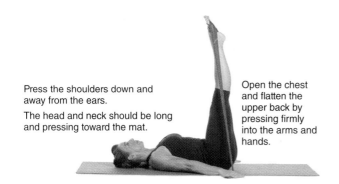

Press the shoulders down and away from the ears.

The head and neck should be long and pressing toward the mat.

Open the chest and flatten the upper back by pressing firmly into the arms and hands.

Level
- ▶ Intermediate

Contraindications
- ▶ Injuries to, pain in, or chronic conditions of the wrists, elbows, knees, hips, or back

Focus
- ▶ Muscles of the arms, legs, core, and upper body

Benefits
- ▶ Strengthens the abdominals and arms
- ▶ Builds upper back flexibility
- ▶ Builds coordination and control

1 Lie on your back. Wrap the band as shown in figure 10.4, page 164. Arms are straight by your sides. Cinch the band so there is slight tension but you can create more as you roll over. To increase or decrease the tension, adjust where you hold the band. Legs are straight and together above the hips, toes pointed. Inhale to prepare.

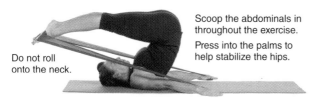

Do not roll onto the neck.

Scoop the abdominals in throughout the exercise.

Press into the palms to help stabilize the hips.

2 Exhale as you press into the hands and roll the hips over the spine until the legs are above the head and parallel to the mat.

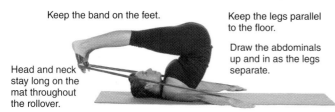

Keep the band on the feet.

Keep the legs parallel to the floor.

Draw the abdominals up and in as the legs separate.

Head and neck stay long on the mat throughout the rollover.

3 Inhale as you separate the legs to sit-bone-distance apart and flex the feet.

4 Exhale as you slowly roll back down the spine until the legs are just above the hips.

5 Inhale as you bring the legs together again and point the toes. Repeat for four to six times and then reverse. To reverse the move, at step 4 keep the legs apart. Inhale as you point the toes. Exhale as you roll the hips back over the spine until they are parallel to the floor. Inhale as you bring the legs together and flex the toes. Exhale as you roll the spine down to bring the legs over the hips. Repeat for four to six times.

Jackknife With the Band

Level
▶ Intermediate to advanced

Contraindications
▶ Injuries to, pain in, or chronic conditions of the wrists, elbows, knees, hips, or back

Focus
▶ Muscles of the arms, legs, core, and upper body

Benefits
▶ Strengthens the abdominals and arms
▶ Builds upper back flexibility
▶ Builds coordination and control
▶ Helps stabilize the shoulders

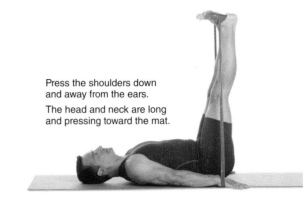

Press the shoulders down and away from the ears.

The head and neck are long and pressing toward the mat.

1 Lie on your back. Wrap the band around your feet with the ends outside the feet. Hold the band under the palms with the ends coming over the thumbs, under the palms, and out on the pinkie side of the hands or with the band over the pinkie side and under the palm. Arms are straight by your sides. Cinch the band so there is slight tension but you can create more as you roll over with the legs. The legs are straight and together above the hips. Inhale to prepare.

Keep the legs straight and the inner thighs pressed together.

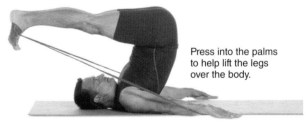

Press into the palms to help lift the legs over the body.

2 Exhale as you roll the lower body off the mat, bringing the legs over the hips and head until they are parallel to the mat.

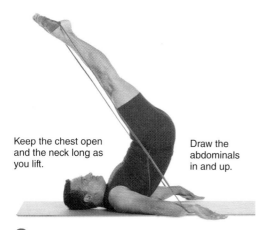

Keep the chest open and the neck long as you lift.

Draw the abdominals in and up.

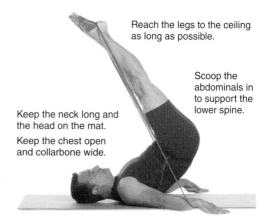

Reach the legs to the ceiling as long as possible.

Scoop the abdominals in to support the lower spine.

Keep the neck long and the head on the mat.

Keep the chest open and collarbone wide.

3 Inhale as you lift the legs toward the ceiling as much as your arms and core allow. Press into the hands to use your arms to lift the body.

4 Exhale as you lower the body slowly and carefully one vertebra at a time. Press into the arms and hands to help control the movement.

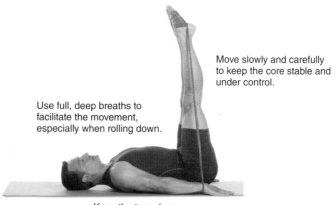

Move slowly and carefully to keep the core stable and under control.

Use full, deep breaths to facilitate the movement, especially when rolling down.

Keep the torso long and straight.

5 Finish the exhale in the start position, legs straight up above your hips and spine flat along the mat, arms by your sides and the band under the palms and over the feet.

6 Inhale as you prepare for the next repetition. Repeat for four to six times, finishing with an inhale.

Control Balance With the Band

Level
▶ Advanced

Contraindications
▶ Injuries to, pain in, or chronic conditions of the wrists, elbows, knees, hips, or back

Focus
▶ Muscles of the arms, legs, core, and upper body

Benefits
▶ Strengthens the abdominals and arms
▶ Builds upper back flexibility
▶ Builds coordination and control
▶ Helps stabilize the shoulders

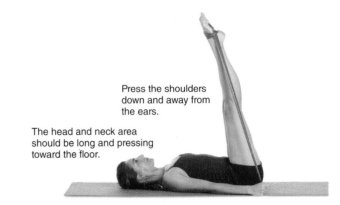

Press the shoulders down and away from the ears.

The head and neck area should be long and pressing toward the floor.

1 Lie on your back. Wrap the band around the feet with the ends out to the sides. Leave some slack in the band between the feet so you can pull the legs apart. Hold the band with a firm grip. Arms are straight by your sides. Cinch the band so there is slight tension but you can create more as you roll over with the legs. Legs are straight and together above the hips. Inhale to prepare.

Keep the legs straight and toes pointed.

Scoop the abdominals in to support the lower spine.

Press into the arms to help lift the legs over the body.

2 Exhale as you roll the lower body off the mat, bringing the legs over the hips and head until they are parallel to the mat.

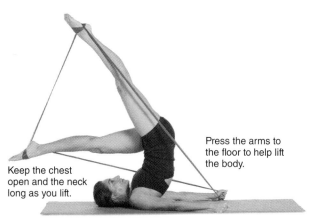

Press the arms to
the floor to help lift
the body.

Keep the chest
open and the neck
long as you lift.

3 Inhale as you lift one leg toward the ceiling as much as your arms, core, and the
band allow. The other leg stays steady, balanced over and parallel to the floor.

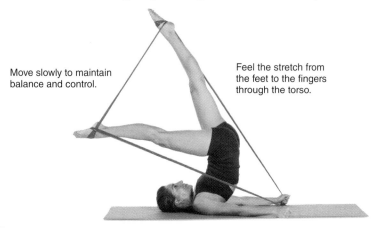

Move slowly to maintain
balance and control.

Feel the stretch from
the feet to the fingers
through the torso.

4 Exhale and scissor the legs, switching them in midair.

5 Inhale and bring the legs together again parallel to the floor. Scoop the abdominals in to support the lower back. Reach through the arms.

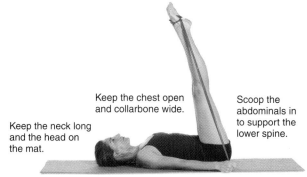

Keep the chest open
and collarbone wide.

Scoop the
abdominals in
to support the
lower spine.

Keep the neck long
and the head on
the mat.

Feel the spine long against the mat.

6 Exhale as you begin to roll down the spine, keeping the legs together and
straight. Finish the exhale in the start position, with the legs straight above the hips
and the spine flat along the mat, arms by your sides with the band under the palms
and over the feet.

Leg Press With the Band

Level

▶ Beginner to intermediate

Contraindications

▶ Injuries to the lower back, knees, ankles, or wrists

Focus

▶ Muscles of the legs, buttocks, and back

Benefits

▶ Increases the strength of the buttocks
▶ Increases leg strength
▶ Increases back strength
▶ Builds balance and coordination

Draw the belly toward the spine.
Keep the arms straight and the upper arms engaged.

The top of the unwrapped foot is on the mat.

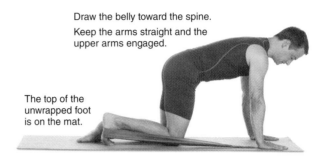

1 Wrap the band around one foot. Start with the middle of the band over the top of the foot, and then wrap the band over and under the foot and out to each side. This secures the band on the foot to prevent slippage. Hold both ends of the band in the hand on the same side as the wrapped foot. Kneel on all fours with your knees directly under your hips and your wrists under the shoulders. The band is underneath the hand holding it. Inhale as you lift the wrapped foot, knee bent. Let the knee hang below the hip with the foot flexed and pointed down.

Feel the leg long and contracted behind the hip.

Keep the foot flexed and reach through the heel.

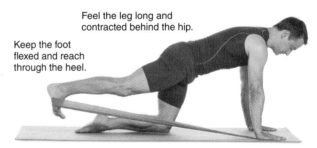

2 Exhale as you extend the leg, bringing the wrapped leg out to just below hip height above the mat. If the tension is too much, grab the ends of the bands closer to the edges.

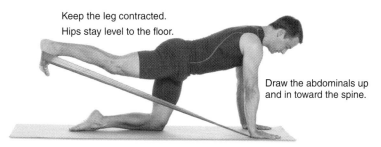

Keep the leg contracted.
Hips stay level to the floor.

Draw the abdominals up
and in toward the spine.

3 Inhale as you lift the straight leg as high as you can without changing the position of the spine or torso.

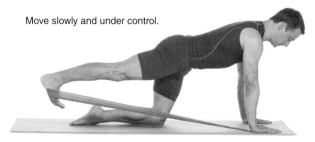

Move slowly and under control.

4 Exhale as you lower the straight, wrapped leg to just below hip height.

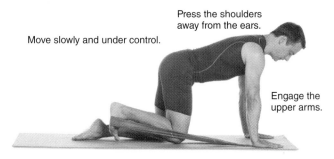

Press the shoulders
away from the ears.

Move slowly and under control.

Engage the
upper arms.

5 Inhale as you bend the knee back to the start position. Repeat for 6 to 10 times. Switch legs and repeat on the other leg for 6 to 10 times.

Swan and Chest Stretch Combo

Level

▶ Intermediate

Contraindications

▶ Injuries to or pain in the lower back, shoulders, elbows, or wrists

Focus

▶ Hamstrings and muscles of the upper back, arms, and shoulders

Benefits

▶ Strengthens the hamstrings, back extensors, and buttocks
▶ Strengthens the arms
▶ Stretches the abdominals and chest
▶ Improves shoulder stability and strength
▶ Improves back extension

Gently squeeze the buttocks to press the pubic bone onto the mat and lengthen the lower spine.

Draw the shoulder blades away from the ears and down the back.

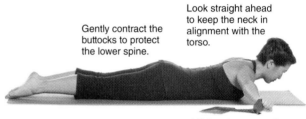

Pull the belly button in toward the spine.

1 Lie on your abdomen with the elbows bent and the hands on the mat in front of and outside of the tops of the shoulders. Place the band under the chest and neck and then over the thumbs and under the palms. Lay your forehead on the mat. Inner thighs are sit-bone-distance apart, with both legs contracted and the belly drawn in away from the mat.

Gently contract the buttocks to protect the lower spine.

Look straight ahead to keep the neck in alignment with the torso.

Lift the sternum and open the chest.

2 Inhale as you press into the hands to straighten the arms and lift the upper body. Lift the head and chest as much as possible without compressing the lower spine.

Feel the abdominals pull in and up, supporting the lower back.

Keep the shoulders away from the ears as the arms reach overhead.

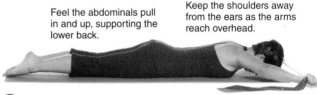

3 Exhale as you lower the upper body to the mat. Reach the arms forward and over the head while holding onto the band.

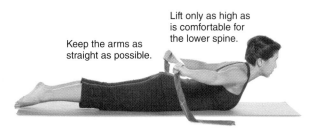

Keep the arms as straight as possible.

Lift only as high as is comfortable for the lower spine.

4 Inhale as you lift the upper body and circle the arms over the head. Bring the band behind the body. Maintain enough laxity in the band so the arm circle is comfortable and doable for the shoulders and scapulae.

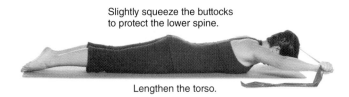

Slightly squeeze the buttocks to protect the lower spine.

Lengthen the torso.

5 Exhale as you circle the arms back up and over the head toward the mat in front of the body as you roll the upper body toward the mat.

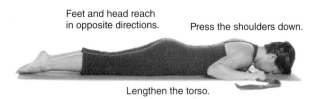

Feet and head reach in opposite directions.

Press the shoulders down.

Lengthen the torso.

6 Inhale as you bend the elbows and bring the hands under and to the side of the shoulders. Exhale to reconnect and prepare for the next repetition. Repeat from step 2 for four to six repetitions.

Side-Lying Series With the Band

Level

► Beginner to intermediate

Contraindications

► Sensitivity in the outer hip area (greater trochanter)
► Pain in, injuries to, or chronic conditions of the hips, neck, shoulders, elbows, wrists, or legs

Focus

► External rotators and muscles of the inner and outer thighs

Benefits

► Promotes control and stability in the hips, pelvis, and torso
► Strengthens the hip, buttock, and lateral thigh muscles

Complete the entire series on one leg, switch sides, and repeat the entire series on the other leg.

LEG LIFT

Feel the waist pull up from the mat and lengthen away from the ribs.

Flex the feet as if standing on them.

1 **Wrap the band over the top of one foot and around so the ends appear beside the foot. Hold onto the band as you lie on your side, torso lined up along the back edge of the mat with the wrapped foot on top. Flex the hips so that the legs are slightly in front of your body. Stack the legs long and straight on top of one another with the toes flexed toward the front. Head lies over the right arm with the palm turned up or down. If you wish, you may bend the right elbow to cradle the head. Bend the top elbow, and place the hand in front of the body for support, placing your hand over the band to hold it securely.**

Gentle Modification

Bend the bottom knee to release any pressure in the lateral bottom leg and greater trochanter area. This modification can be used for any of the side-lying exercises.

Keep the torso in a straight line.

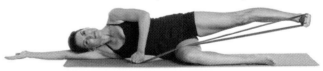

Keep the bottom knee in front of the hip.

Challenge

Prop up the head with the bottom hand, and slightly lift the bottom rib cage off the mat. If you feel strain in your neck or shoulder, return to the original start position or use the gentle modification.

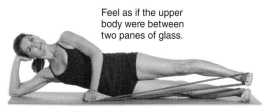

Feel as if the upper body were between two panes of glass.

The body should feel long and strong like a board.

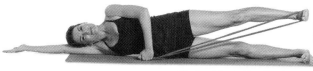

Flex at the hip, not at the waist.

Feel the leg reach away from the hip as it lifts.

Contract the bottom leg to help balance the body.

2 Inhale as you lift the top leg off the bottom leg to hip height or just slightly above.

3 Exhale as you lower the leg to rest on top of the bottom leg. Maintain the length in the torso as you lift and lower the leg. Keep both legs strong and activated. Repeat for 8 to 10 repetitions on this leg, and then go to the Knee Press on this side.

KNEE PRESS

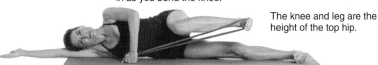

Keep the waist long and cinched in as you bend the knee.

The knee and leg are the height of the top hip.

4 Inhale as you bend the top knee in as far as the hip.

5 Exhale as you straighten the top leg and bring it just above the bottom leg. Repeat for 8 to 10 repetitions on this leg, and then go to the Circle on this side.

CIRCLE

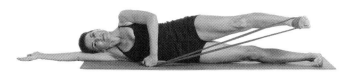

6 Inhale as you bring the top leg forward and up, creating a half circle in front of the body.

7 Exhale as you bring the top leg back and down, creating a half circle behind the body. Circles are small and contained, the size of a dinner plate. Shoulders, torso, and hips are aligned and stacked on top of one another. Repeat for 8 to 10 repetitions, circling in a forward direction. Reverse direction and repeat for another 8 to 10 repetitions, and then go to the Leg Kick on this side.

(continued)

Side-Lying Series With the Band *(continued)*

LEG KICK

Use the top hand to
stabilize and control
the movement.

Keep the waist long
as you kick forward.

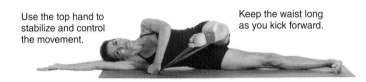

8 Inhale twice with a double pulse as you kick the top leg forward as far as possible without changing the position of the torso and waist.

Keep the upper body from
leaning too far forward as
you kick back.

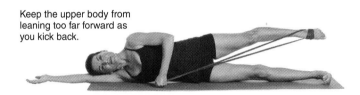

9 Exhale with a smooth breath as you kick the leg back. Repeat from step 8 for five to seven repetitions. Switch the band to the other leg and repeat the entire series, beginning with Leg Lift, on the other leg.

Chapter 11

Pilates Routines

The Pilates routines described in this chapter are drawn from the individual exercises discussed in chapters 2 through 10. In the routines, you will combine moves to create an individual program designed to help you achieve a certain goal. Routines vary in length from 10 to 40 minutes or more. Depending on your goals and skill level, you may want to combine routines to suit your needs. Routines are labeled with the level of skill required so you can appropriately choose the program or series of programs right for you.

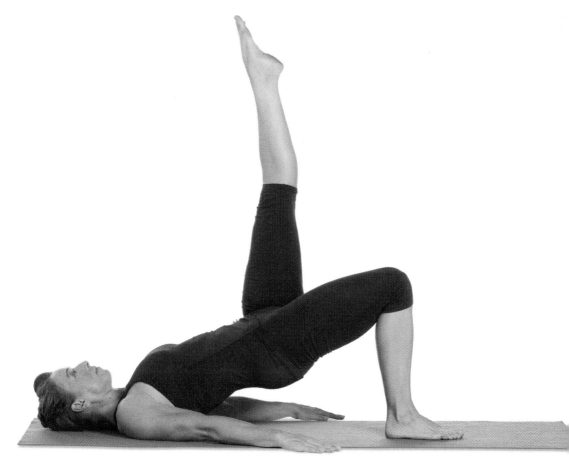

Most of the routines begin from a standing position. I have chosen this position because it is the easiest one for most people to get into and the position that places the least amount of stress on the body. (People with joint issues or who lack flexibility may have difficulty sitting or lying on the mat.) Standing is also an easy position for people to start to build awareness of their bodies and to see themselves in a mirror if need be.

These routines provide a sequence or flow to your Pilates practice that will allow you to connect your breath with continuous movement. This rhythm is integral in a true Pilates practice as it creates smooth, graceful, and functional movement patterns. Movements practiced this way place less stress on the joints and provide the most efficient way of moving the body.

The first four Pilates routines (pages 191 to 197) focus on stretching, relaxing, and lengthening the body. They target the hips, legs, shoulders, and lower back. These are some of the more common areas where stress resides, thus lessening the overall range of motion and flexibility of the body in general. These routines are aimed at the beginner but are a good warm-up for the seasoned Pilates student as well.

Good posture is a key element to feeling and looking good. Bad posture causes common ailments such as back and neck pain. Since posture is the most essential element of everyday movement mechanics, it is a great place to start working in a general exercise regimen. The next three routines (pages 198 to 204) target the key muscles that factor into maintaining good posture. These programs will help you perfect your posture or correct common causes for poor posture. These programs can be used daily by themselves, or they can be combined with other routines to create a longer, more complete workout.

For a quick pick-me-up or to focus on losing weight, try the next two Pilates routines (pages 205 through 210) to energize and revitalize your workouts. In 10 to 20 minutes, they provide the power and punch you need to reduce your body or build lean muscles. The secret key to these workouts is the pace; you will move quickly between exercises without stopping, providing a cardio effect that will invigorate any program.

The next four routines (pages 211 through 217) use traditional Pilates movements and props such as the stability ball, Pilates ring, and stretch band to infuse a challenge to the core, coordination, flexibility, and strength. These routines are sure to provide a powerful and strong workout for intermediate to advanced Pilates practitioners.

The final four workouts (pages 218 through 228) combine advanced exercises with a faster pace and no breaks. These are very tough workouts. From Total Body Strength, which focuses on strengthening the entire body, to three routines that target a specific region of the body, these workouts will challenge even the most proficient student.

Restore Flexibility

The exercises in this routine provide an avenue for opening up the tight areas of the body. This is a full-body flexibility routine that also provides a great warm-up for more challenging routines. Since flexibility helps with overall range of motion and, ultimately, good posture, this routine can be done daily to restore elasticity and range of motion in tense areas of the body.

LEVEL: Beginner
LENGTH: 10 to 15 minutes

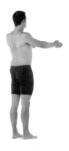
Shoulder Warming, page 13

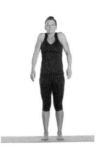
Shoulder Shrug, page 24

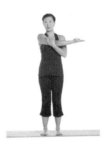
Arm Stretch, page 16

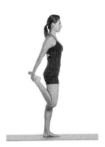
Leg Stretch, page 18

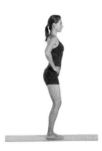
Pelvic Clock, page 20

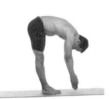
Roll-Down, page 22

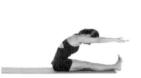
Roll-Up, page 66

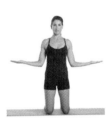
External Rotation With Arms, page 27

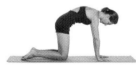
Cat-Cow, page 30

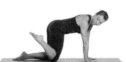
Tail Wag, page 31

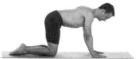
Sternum Drop, page 32

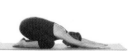
Child's Pose, page 26

(continued)

Restore Flexibility

(continued)

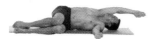

Pinwheel, page 38

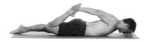

Thigh Stretch, page 49

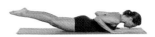

Swan, page 54

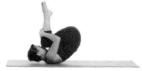

Rolling Like a Ball,
page 97

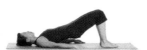

Pelvic Peel, page 62

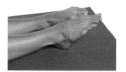

Footwork Series,
page 94

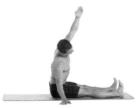

**Spine Stretch: Forward
and Side,** page 90

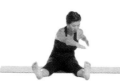

Saw, page 102

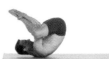

Seal, page 104

Energy in the A.M.

A few moments of exercise in the morning can do wonders for picking up your energy level. This workout will provide you with plenty of energy throughout the day in a mere 10 minutes. Although titled Energy in the A.M., this workout can be done at any time throughout the day to provide a little pick-me-up. Perform the exercises rhythmically, moving from one exercise to the next with precision and concentration. Try not to take a break between exercises.

LEVEL: Beginner
LENGTH: 10 minutes

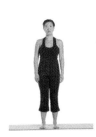

Modified Pilates Stance,
page 12

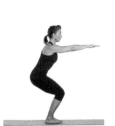

Heel Raise With Squat,
page 14

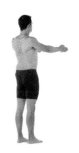

Shoulder Warming,
page 13

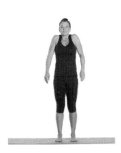

Shoulder Shrug,
page 24

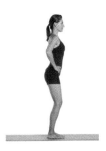

Pelvic Clock, page 20

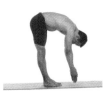

Roll-Down, page 22

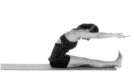

Roll-Up, page 66

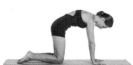

Cat-Cow, page 30

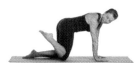

Tail Wag, page 31

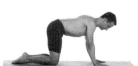

Sternum Drop, page 32

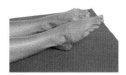

Footwork Series,
page 94

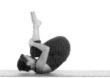

Rolling Like a Ball,
page 97

(continued)

Energy in the A.M.

(continued)

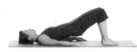

Pelvic Peel, page 62

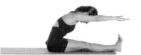

Roll-Up, page 66

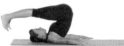

Rollover, page 78

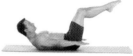

Hundred, page 64

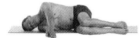

Pinwheel (right),
page 38

Swimming, page 51

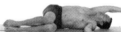

Pinwheel (left),
page 38

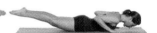

Swan, page 54

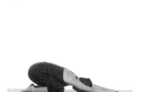

Child's Pose, page 26

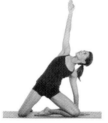

Mermaid, page 92

Seal, page 104

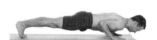

Push-Up, page 55

P.M. Relaxation

These exercises are a great way to prepare the body to rest and relax in the evening. They also can be used for a warm-up before another routine. Move slowly and under control, working methodically from one exercise to the next. If you are using this routine to prepare for rest, work with the thought of keeping the heart rate down.

LEVEL: Beginner
LENGTH: 10 minutes

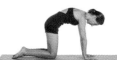

Cat-Cow, page 30

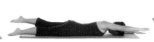

Oppositional Stretch, page 48

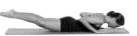

Swan, page 54

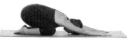

Child's Pose, page 26

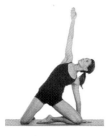

Mermaid, page 92

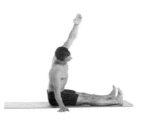

Spine Stretch: Forward and Side, page 90

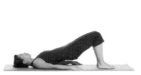

Pelvic Peel, page 62

Stress Release

Relieving stress daily is important for overall good health and happiness. Take a few minutes each day to open the joints, move the body, and stretch the muscles to relieve stress and calm your body and mind. This routine can be done daily as a warm-up for another routine or activity.

LEVEL: Beginner
LENGTH: 15 to 20 minutes

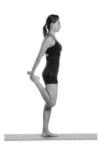

Heel Raise With Squat,
page 14

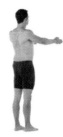

Shoulder Warming,
page 13

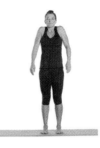

Shoulder Shrug,
page 24

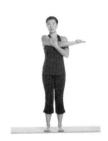

Arm Stretch, page 16

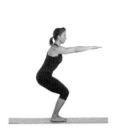

Leg Stretch, page 18

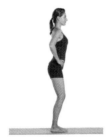

Pelvic Clock, page 20

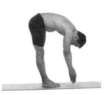

Roll-Down, page 22

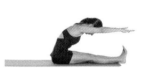

Roll-Up, page 66

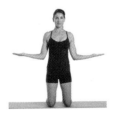

External Rotation With Arms, page 27

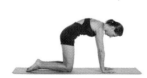

Cat-Cow, page 30

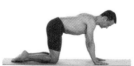

Sternum Drop, page 32

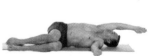

Pinwheel, page 38

Stress Release

(continued)

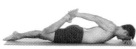

Thigh Stretch, page 49

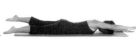

Oppositional Stretch, page 48

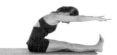

Roll-Up, page 66

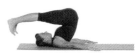

Rollover, page 78

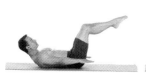

Hundred, page 64

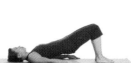

Pelvic Peel, page 62

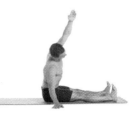

Spine Stretch: Forward and Side, page 90

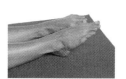

Footwork Series, page 94

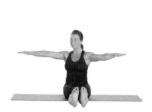

Spine Twist, page 100

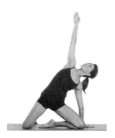

Mermaid, page 92

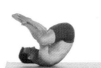

Seal, page 104

Modified Lower Back Core Focus

This program focuses on strengthening the core, specifically the lower back. A weak lower back frequently causes pain and poor posture, leading to muscular imbalance and possibly other issues and pain. A strong lower back provides a better base for more challenging work and exercise and will allow you to stand straighter and taller. This program can be used as a warm-up before other programs or can stand on its own as an efficient way to warm up and strengthen the lower back, an integral part of the core that promotes better posture and a stronger body.

LEVEL: Beginner
LENGTH: 10 to 15 minutes

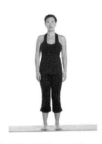
Modified Pilates Stance, page 12

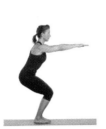
Heel Raise With Squat, page 14

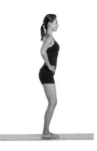
Pelvic Clock, page 20

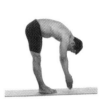
Roll-Down, page 22

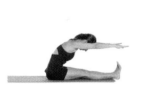
Roll-Up, page 66

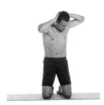
Oblique Crunch, page 28

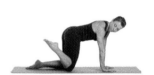
Tail Wag, page 31

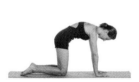
Cat-Cow, page 30

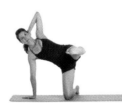
Kneeling Side Kick, page 33

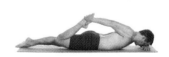
Thigh Stretch, page 49

Modified Lower Back Core Focus

(continued)

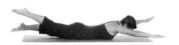

Swimming, page 51

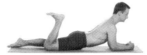

Single-Leg Kick,
page 50

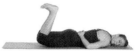

Double-Leg Kick,
page 52

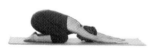

Child's Pose, page 26

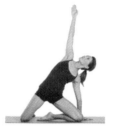

Mermaid, page 92

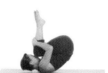

Rolling Like a Ball,
page 97

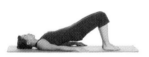

Pelvic Peel, page 62

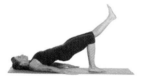

Shoulder Bridge,
page 76

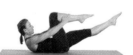

Single-Leg Stretch,
page 68

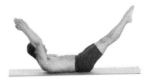

Double-Leg Stretch,
page 70

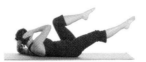

Crisscross, page 73

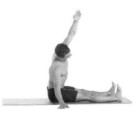

**Spine Stretch: Forward
and Side,** page 90

Core Concentration

This routine focuses on strengthening the entire core from top to bottom and front to back. A strong core leads to a strong body, which leads to good and correct posture. Someone with a weak core is unable to hold herself up correctly. Strengthening the entire core provides a solid base to support the muscles and bones in a way that does not stress the joints. Use this program daily to strengthen your core and correct your posture. It also can be combined with other programs.

LEVEL: Beginner to intermediate
LENGTH: 15 to 20 minutes

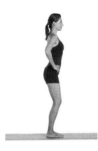

Pelvic Clock, page 20

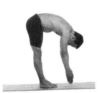

Roll-Down, page 22

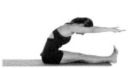

Roll-Up, page 66

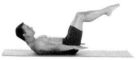

Hundred, page 64

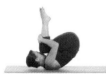

Rolling Like a Ball, page 97

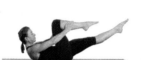

Single-Leg Stretch, page 68

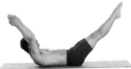

Double-Leg Stretch, page 70

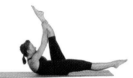

Single Straight-Leg Stretch, page 71

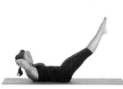

Double Straight-Leg Stretch, page 72

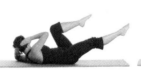

Crisscross, page 73

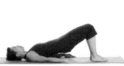

Pelvic Peel, page 62

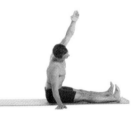

Spine Stretch: Forward and Side, page 90

Core Concentration

(continued)

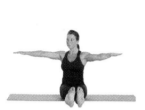

Spine Twist, page 100

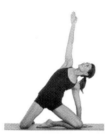

Mermaid, page 92

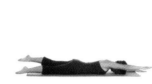

Oppositional Stretch,
page 48

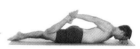

Thigh Stretch, page 49

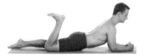

Single-Leg Kick,
page 50

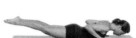

Swan, page 54

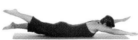

Swimming, page 51

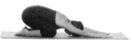

Child's Pose, page 26

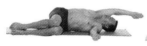

Pinwheel, page 38

Leg Lift, page 39

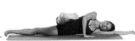

Front Kick, page 41

Seal, page 104

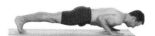

Push-Up, page 55

Better Posture

Keeping your posture at its best can be quite difficult these days. People often drive too much, sit too much, stand too much, and all with poor posture. Poor posture may lead to pain or weakness, but correcting it can be very difficult. This program may be used daily or weekly as long as you use it. The program is challenging but doable and should be done at least every other day.

LEVEL: Beginner to intermediate

LENGTH: 15 to 20 minutes

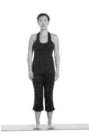

Modified Pilates Stance,
page 12

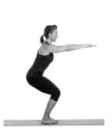

Heel Raise With Squat,
page 14

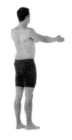

Shoulder Warming,
page 13

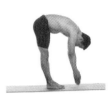

Roll-Down, page 22

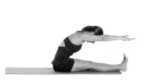

Roll-Up, page 66

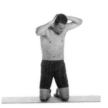

Oblique Crunch,
page 28

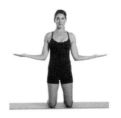

External Rotation With Arms, page 27

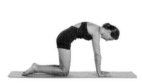

Cat-Cow, page 30

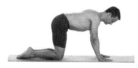

Sternum Drop, page 32

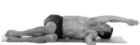

Pinwheel, page 38

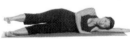

Leg Lift, page 39

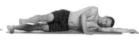

Side-Lying Leg Circle,
page 40

Better Posture

(continued)

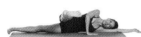

Front Kick, page 41

Leg Tap, page 42

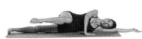

Side-Lying Bicycle,
page 44

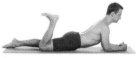

Single-Leg Kick,
page 50

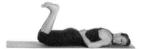

Double-Leg Kick,
page 52

Swan, page 54

Swimming, page 51

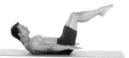

Hundred, page 64

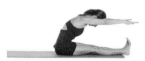

Roll-Up, page 66

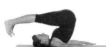

Rollover, page 78

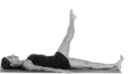

Supine Leg Circle,
page 60

Rolling Like a Ball,
page 97

(continued)

Better Posture

(continued)

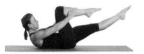

Single-Leg Stretch,
page 68

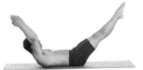

Double-Leg Stretch,
page 70

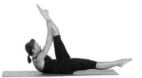

**Single Straight-Leg
Stretch,** page 71

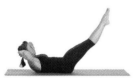

**Double Straight-Leg
Stretch,** page 72

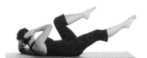

Crisscross, page 73

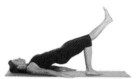

Shoulder Bridge,
page 76

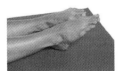

Footwork Series,
page 94

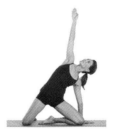

Mermaid, page 92

Simple Weight-Loss Pilates

This workout focuses on burning calories to help you lose weight. To burn calories, you must work rhythmically, moving from one exercise to the next with ease and not stopping to take a break if at all possible. This does not mean moving as fast as you can. It means moving with control, concentration, and precision at a somewhat faster pace than normal and going from one exercise to the next with little or no break. Focus on form and quality versus speed and quantity to get the desired effects of this workout.

LEVEL: Beginner to intermediate
LENGTH: 30 to 45 minutes

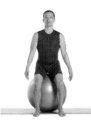

Bouncing in Place,
page 111

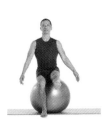

Bouncing While Kicking,
page 112

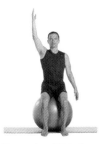

Bouncing With Arm Raised, page 113

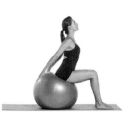

Pelvic Clock With Stretching on the Ball,
page 114

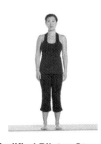

Modified Pilates Stance,
page 12

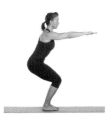

Heel Raise With Squat,
page 14

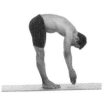

Roll-Down, page 22

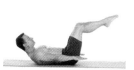

Hundred, page 64

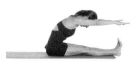

Roll-Up, page 66

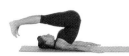

Rollover, page 78

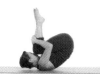

Rolling Like a Ball,
page 97

(continued)

Simple Weight-Loss Pilates

(continued)

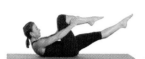

Single-Leg Stretch,
page 68

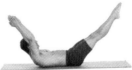

Double-Leg Stretch,
page 70

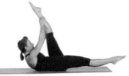

**Single Straight-Leg
Stretch,** page 71

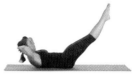

**Double Straight-Leg
Stretch,** page 72

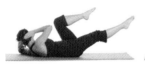

Crisscross, page 73

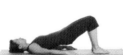

Pelvic Peel, page 62

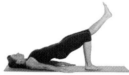

Shoulder Bridge,
page 76

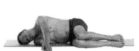

Pinwheel (right),
page 38

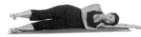

Leg Lift (right),
page 39

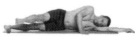

**Side-Lying Leg Circle
(right),** page 40

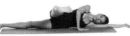

Front Kick (right),
page 41

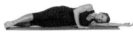

Leg Tap (right),
page 42

Simple Weight-Loss Pilates

(continued)

Side-Lying Bicycle (right), page 44

Oppositional Stretch, page 48

Swimming, page 51

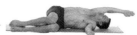

Pinwheel (left), page 38

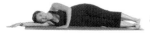

Leg Lift (left), page 39

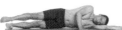

Side-Lying Leg Circle (left), page 40

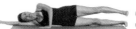

Front Kick (left), page 41

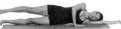

Leg Tap (left), page 42

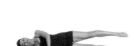

Side-Lying Bicycle (left), page 44

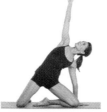

Mermaid, page 92

Seal, page 104

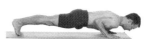

Push-Up, page 55

Long and Lean Muscles

This workout is quick and easy yet focused and direct. You will achieve the desired results if you complete this workout in a focused and precise way and move from one exercise to the next without a break. Think of lengthening out and working from one end point to the other as you move each limb and muscle. Concentrate on the precise movement of each exercise as you move from exercise to exercise.

LEVEL: Intermediate

LENGTH: 10 to 15 minutes

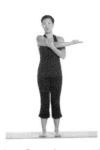

Arm Stretch, page 16

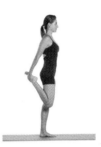

Leg Stretch, page 18

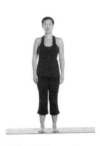

Modified Pilates Stance,
page 12

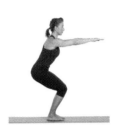

Heel Raise With Squat,
page 14

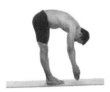

Roll-Down, page 22

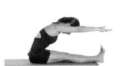

Roll-Up, page 66

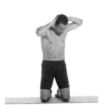

Oblique Crunch,
page 28

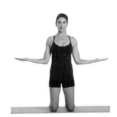

**External Rotation With
Arms,** page 27

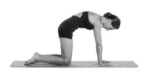

Cat-Cow, page 30

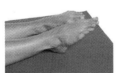

Footwork Series,
page 94

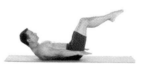

Hundred, page 64

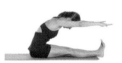

Roll-Up, page 66

Long and Lean Muscles

(continued)

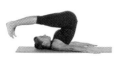

Rollover, page 78

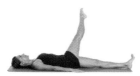

Supine Leg Circle,
page 60

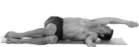

Pinwheel, page 38

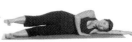

Leg Lift, page 39

Side-Lying Leg Circle,
page 40

Front Kick, page 41

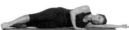

Leg Tap, page 42

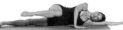

Side-Lying Bicycle,
page 44

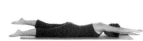

Oppositional Stretch,
page 48

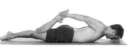

Thigh Stretch, page 49

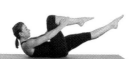

Single-Leg Stretch,
page 68

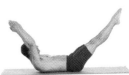

Double-Leg Stretch,
page 70

(continued)

Long and Lean Muscles

(continued)

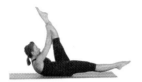

Single Straight-Leg Stretch, page 71

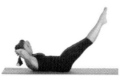

Double Straight-Leg Stretch, page 72

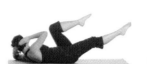

Crisscross, page 73

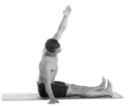

Spine Stretch: Forward and Side, page 90

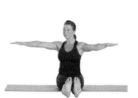

Spine Twist, page 100

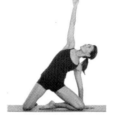

Mermaid, page 92

Seal, page 104

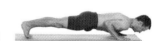

Push-Up, page 55

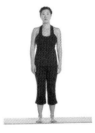

Modified Pilates Stance, page 12

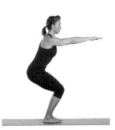

Heel Raise With Squat, page 14

Get on the Ball

This stability ball workout is challenging and demands that you push your levels of coordination and core strength to the max. Fluidly move from one exercise to the next, but take the time to set up the ball and your body properly so you can perform the move correctly.

LEVEL: Intermediate to advanced
LENGTH: 10 to 15 minutes

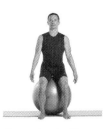
Bouncing in Place,
page 111

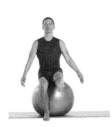
Bouncing While Kicking,
page 112

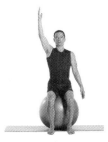
Bouncing With Arm Raised, page 113

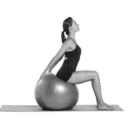
Pelvic Clock With Stretching on the Ball,
page 114

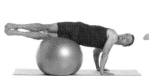
Side Rollover on the Ball,
page 136

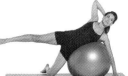
Side-Lying Leg Lift on the Ball (right), page 133

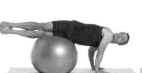
Side Rollover on the Ball,
page 136

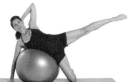
Side-Lying Leg Lift on the Ball (left), page 133

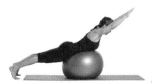
Swan on the Ball,
page 128

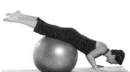
Push-Up on the Ball,
page 132

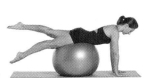
Swimming on the Ball,
page 129

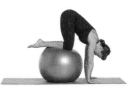
Pike Variations on the Ball, page 130

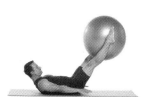
Hundred With the Ball,
page 122

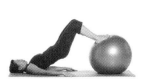
Bridging Variations on the Ball, page 120

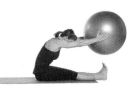
Roll-Up Variations With the Ball, page 116

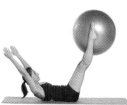
Rollover Pass the Ball,
page 118

Pilates Ring for Muscle Tone

For this workout, you will use the Pilates ring. This routine will challenge and tone your body. Thoroughly complete each exercise, and when moving from one exercise to the next, take only the time necessary to set up the exercise. This workout might be short, but it's thorough. It is a great routine on its own or combined with any of the other workouts in this book.

LEVEL: Intermediate to advanced
LENGTH: 10 minutes

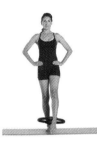

Standing Single-Leg Series: Front, Side, and Back, page 140

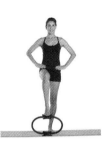

Standing Single-Leg Series: Balance, page 139

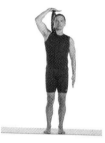

Standing Arm Series, page 142

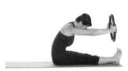

Roll-Up With the Ring, page 144

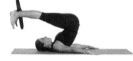

Rollover With the Ring, page 146

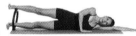

Side-Lying Top Leg Press Down With the Ring (right), page 156

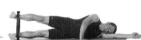

Side-Lying Top Leg Press Up With the Ring (right), page 157

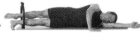

Side-Lying Leg Circle With the Ring (right), page 158

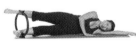

Side-Lying Bicycle With the Ring (right), page 159

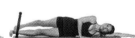

Leg Tap With the Ring (right), page 160

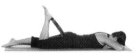

Single-Leg Press (right and left), page 155

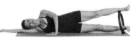

Side-Lying Top Leg Press Down With the Ring (left), page 156

Pilates Ring for Muscle Tone

(continued)

Side-Lying Top Leg Press Up With the Ring (left), page 157

Side-Lying Leg Circle With the Ring (left), page 158

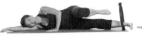

Side-Lying Bicycle With the Ring (left), page 159

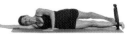

Leg Tap With the Ring (left), page 160

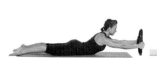

Swan With the Ring, page 154

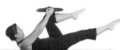

Single-Leg Stretch With the Ring, page 148

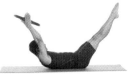

Double-Leg Stretch With the Ring, page 149

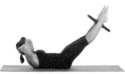

Double Straight-Leg Stretch With the Ring, page 150

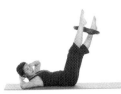

Crisscross With the Ring, page 151

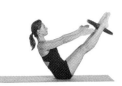

Teaser Variations With the Ring, page 152

Total Body Band

This stretch band workout is short but effective. It works well on its own or as an addition to another workout. When working through the exercises, be sure to follow the directions for holding the band. Set up each exercise with precision and ease so that you can work rhythmically from one exercise to the next. This will give a flow to the workout and add to its effectiveness.

LEVEL: Intermediate to advanced
LENGTH: 10 minutes

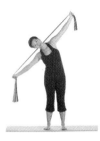

Standing Stretches With the Band, page 166

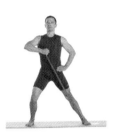

Side Arm Lunge Series, page 168

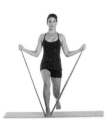

Double-Arm Lunge Series, page 170

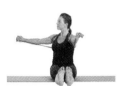

Spine Twist With the Band, page 172

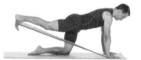

Leg Press With the Band, page 182

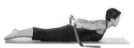

Swan and Chest Stretch Combo, page 184

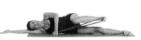

Side-Lying Series With the Band (right and left), page 186

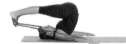

Rollover With the Band, page 177

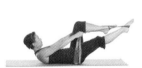

Single-Leg Stretch With the Band, page 173

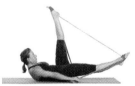

Single Straight-Leg Stretch With the Band, page 174

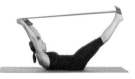

Double-Leg Stretch With the Band, page 175

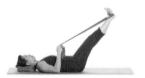

Diamond Leg Press, page 176

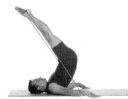

Jackknife With the Band, page 178

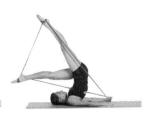

Control Balance With the Band, page 180

Props Complete Strength

This workout combines most of the exercises from chapters 8, 9, and 10 into a flowing, smooth, intelligent, and very challenging workout. Be prepared to work hard and sweat! You will work the entire body and use all three pieces of equipment in a flowing, rhythmic manner. Take your time when moving from one exercise to the next and when changing equipment. Have all three pieces close by so you can move quickly from one piece to the next.

LEVEL: Advanced

LENGTH: 20 to 30 minutes

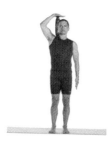

Standing Arm Series,
page 142

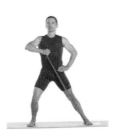

Side Arm Lunge Series,
page 168

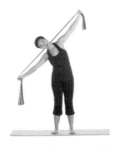

Standing Stretches With the Band, page 166

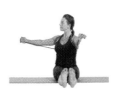

Spine Twist With the Band, page 172

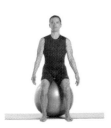

Bouncing in Place,
page 111

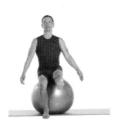

Bouncing While Kicking,
page 112

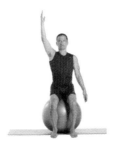

Bouncing With Arm Raised, page 113

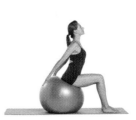

Pelvic Clock With Stretching on the Ball,
page 114

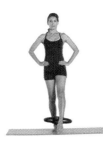

Standing Single-Leg Series: Front, Side, and Back, page 140

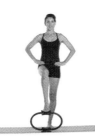

Standing Single-Leg Series: Balance,
page 139

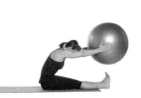

Roll-Up Variations With the Ball, page 116

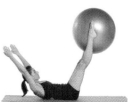

Rollover Pass the Ball,
page 118

(continued)

Props Complete Strength

(continued)

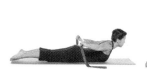

Swan and Chest Stretch Combo, page 184

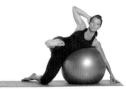

Side-Lying Front Leg Kick on the Ball (right), page 135

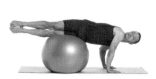

Side Rollover on the Ball, page 136

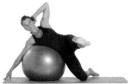

Side-Lying Front Leg Kick on the Ball (left), page 135

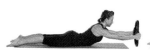

Swan With the Ring, page 154

Single-Leg Press, page 155

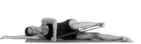

Side-Lying Series With the Band (right and left), page 186

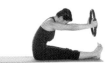

Roll-Up With the Ring, page 144

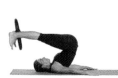

Rollover With the Ring, page 146

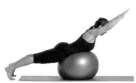

Swan on the Ball, page 128

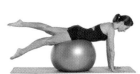

Swimming on the Ball, page 129

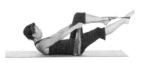

Single-Leg Stretch With the Band, page 173

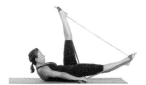

Single Straight-Leg Stretch With the Band, page 174

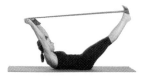

Double-Leg Stretch With the Band, page 175

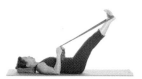

Diamond Leg Press, page 176

Props Complete Strength

(continued)

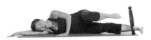

Side-Lying Bicycle With the Ring (right and left), page 159

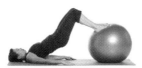

Bridging Variations on the Ball, page 120

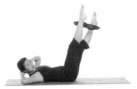

Crisscross With the Ring, page 151

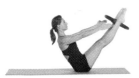

Teaser Variations With the Ring, page 152

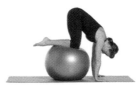

Pike Variations on the Ball, page 130

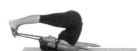

Rollover With the Band, page 177

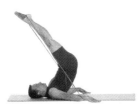

Jackknife With the Band, page 178

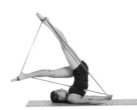

Control Balance With the Band, page 180

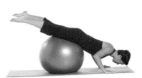

Push-Up on the Ball, page 132

Total Body Strength

This routine is a head-to-toe full-body workout that will challenge even the most advanced Pilates student. Once mastered, it can be done in 20 minutes; until then, work through each exercise with precision and accuracy, taking your time to complete each exercise correctly. Each time you do the routine, move a bit faster, reducing the time between exercises so you flow with ease from one exercise to the next.

LEVEL: Intermediate to advanced

LENGTH: Approximately 20 to 30 minutes

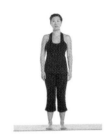

Modified Pilates Stance,
page 12

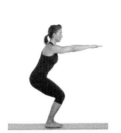

Heel Raise With Squat,
page 14

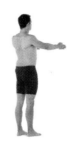

Shoulder Warming,
page 13

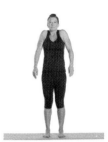

Shoulder Shrug,
page 24

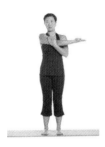

Arm Stretch, page 16

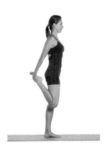

Leg Stretch, page 18

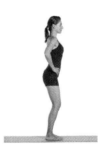

Pelvic Clock, page 20

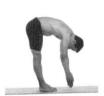

Roll-Down, page 22

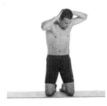

Oblique Crunch,
page 28

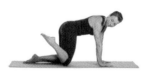

Tail Wag, page 31

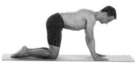

Sternum Drop, page 32

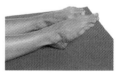

Footwork Series,
page 94

Total Body Strength

(continued)

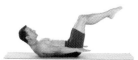

Hundred, page 64

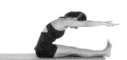

Roll-Up, page 66

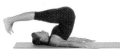

Rollover, page 78

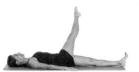

Supine Leg Circle,
page 60

Rolling Like a Ball,
page 97

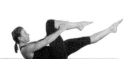

Single-Leg Stretch,
page 68

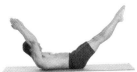

Double-Leg Stretch,
page 70

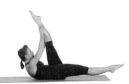

**Single Straight-Leg
Stretch,** page 71

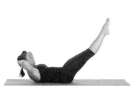

**Double Straight-Leg
Stretch,** page 72

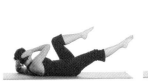

Crisscross, page 73

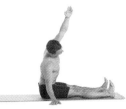

**Spine Stretch: Forward
and Side,** page 90

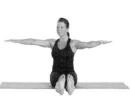

Spine Twist, page 100

(continued)

Total Body Strength

(continued)

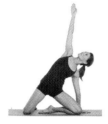
Mermaid (right),
page 92

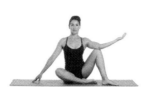
Side Bend (right),
page 98

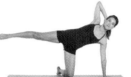
**Kneeling Side Kick
(right),** page 33

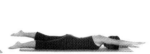
Oppositional Stretch,
page 48

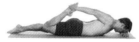
Thigh Stretch,
page 49

Swimming, page 51

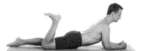
Single-Leg Kick,
page 50

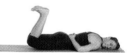
Double-Leg Kick,
page 52

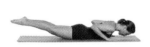
Swan, page 54

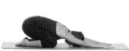
Child's Pose, page 26

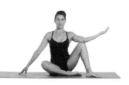
Mermaid (left), page 92

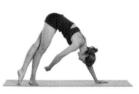
Side Bend (left), page 98

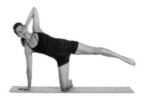
Kneeling Side Kick (left),
page 33

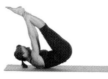
Open Leg Rocker,
page 99

Corkscrew, page 79

Total Body Strength

(continued)

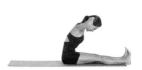

Neck Pull, page 81

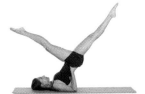

Scissors, page 83

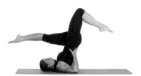

Bicycle, page 85

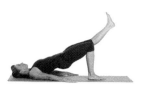

Shoulder Bridge,
page 76

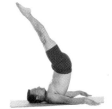

Jackknife, page 87

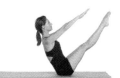

Teaser, page 74

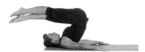

Boomerang, page 105

Seal, page 104

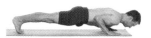

Push-Up, page 55

Upper Body Focus

Although this workout focuses on the upper body, it requires correct breathing, core control, and focused concentration on each move. It can be used as a stand-alone workout or added to another routine in this book to create a longer full-body workout.

LEVEL: Intermediate to advanced
LENGTH: 15 minutes

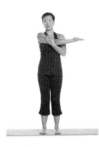

Arm Stretch, page 16

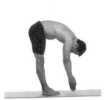

Roll-Down, page 22

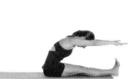

Roll-Up, page 66

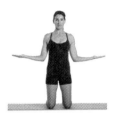

External Rotation With Arms, page 27

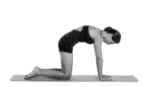

Cat-Cow, page 30

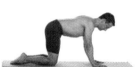

Sternum Drop, page 32

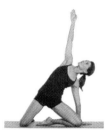

Mermaid, page 92

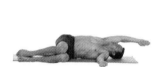

Pinwheel, page 38

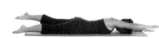

Oppositional Stretch, page 48

Swimming, page 51

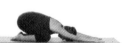

Child's Pose, page 26

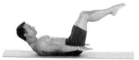

Hundred, page 64

Rolling Like a Ball, page 97

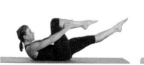

Single-Leg Stretch, page 68

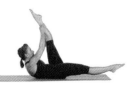

Single Straight-Leg Stretch, page 71

Upper Body Focus

(continued)

Corkscrew, page 79

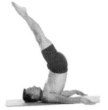

Jackknife, page 87

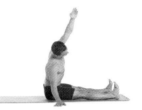

Spine Stretch: Forward and Side, page 90

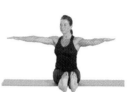

Spine Twist, page 100

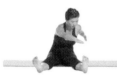

Saw, page 102

Open Leg Rocker, page 99

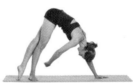

Side Bend, page 98

Seal, page 104

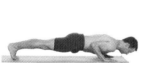

Push-Up, page 55

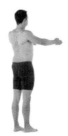

Shoulder Warming, page 13

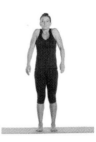

Shoulder Shrug, page 24

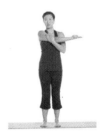

Arm Stretch, page 16

Lower Body Focus

This workout concentrates on the muscles of the lower body but also incorporates the core muscles and upper body. This routine can be used alone or combined with another routine to create a complete longer workout. Move carefully and methodically through each exercise to gain the full benefits, and then work on picking up the pace to add rhythm and flow.

LEVEL: Intermediate to advanced
LENGTH: 15 minutes

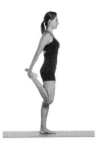

Leg Stretch, page 18

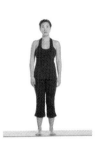

Modified Pilates Stance, page 12

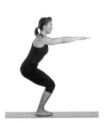

Heel Raise With Squat, page 14

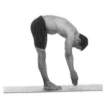

Roll-Down, page 22

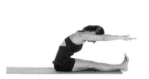

Roll-Up, page 66

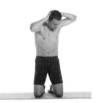

Oblique Crunch, page 28

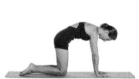

Cat-Cow, page 30

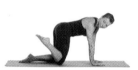

Tail Wag, page 31

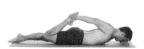

Thigh Stretch, page 49

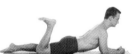

Single-Leg Kick, page 50

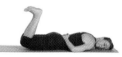

Double-Leg Kick, page 52

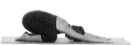

Child's Pose, page 26

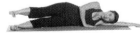

Leg Lift, page 39

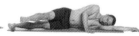

Side-Lying Leg Circle, page 40

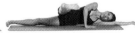

Front Kick, page 41

Leg Tap,
page 42

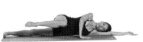

Side-Lying Bicycle,
page 44

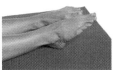

Footwork Series,
page 94

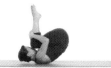

Rolling Like a Ball,
page 97

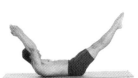

Double-Leg Stretch,
page 70

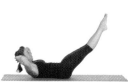

**Double Straight-Leg
Stretch,** page 72

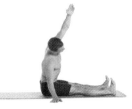

**Spine Stretch: Forward
and Side,** page 90

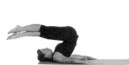

Boomerang,
page 105

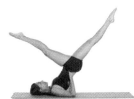

Scissors, page 83

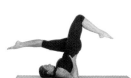

Bicycle, page 85

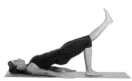

Shoulder Bridge, page 76

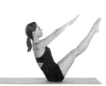

Teaser, page 74

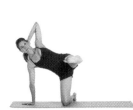

Kneeling Side Kick,
page 33

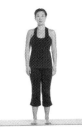

Modified Pilates Stance,
page 12

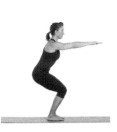

Heel Raise With Squat,
page 14

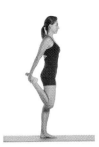

Leg Stretch,
page 18

Core Focus

This core-focused routine is based on the original 34 exercises developed by Joseph Pilates. Not all of the original 34 exercises are included here, and there are a few movements that were not included in the original 34 exercises. Since Pilates is based on using the core effectively, this workout will help you focus on the core to strengthen it. Once mastered, this program can be done daily, either on its own or in conjunction with another routine.

LEVEL: Advanced
LENGTH: 20 to 30 minutes

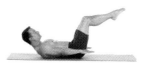
Hundred, page 64

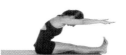
Roll-Up, page 66

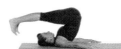
Rollover, page 78

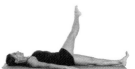
Supine Leg Circle, page 60

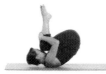
Rolling Like a Ball, page 97

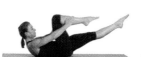
Single-Leg Stretch, page 68

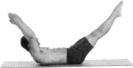
Double-Leg Stretch, page 70

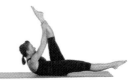
Single Straight-Leg Stretch, page 71

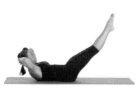
Double Straight-Leg Stretch, page 72

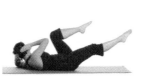
Crisscross, page 73

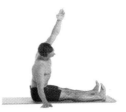
Spine Stretch: Forward and Side, page 90

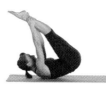
Open Leg Rocker, page 99

Core Focus

(continued)

Corkscrew, page 79

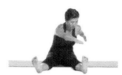

Saw, page 102

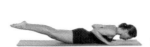

Swan, page 54

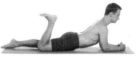

Single-Leg Kick, page 50

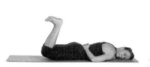

Double-Leg Kick, page 52

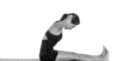

Neck Pull, page 81

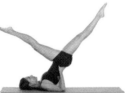

Scissors, page 83

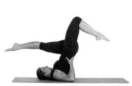

Bicycle, page 85

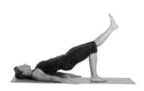

Shoulder Bridge, page 76

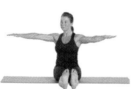

Spine Twist, page 100

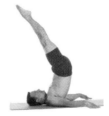

Jackknife, page 87

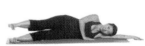

Leg Lift, page 39

(continued)

Core Focus

(continued)

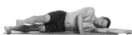 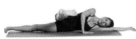 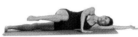 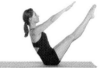

Side-Lying Leg Circle,
page 40

Front Kick, page 41

Side-Lying Bicycle,
page 44

Teaser, page 74

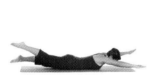 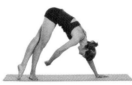 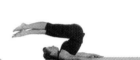

Swimming, page 51

Kneeling Side Kick,
page 33

Side Bend, page 98

Boomerang, page 105

 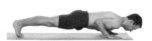

Seal, page 104

Push-Up, page 55

About the Author

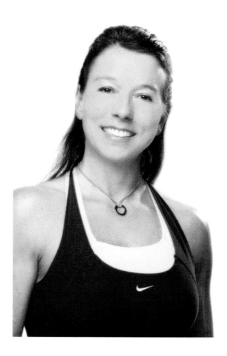

Portia Page is a Pilates instructor at Propel Pilates and Fitness in Rancho Bernardo, California. She is a gold-certified Pilates teacher through Pilates Method Alliance (PMA), a faculty member of Balanced Body University (BBU), and a Stott Pilates-certified instructor of levels 1 and 2. She was also a master instructor with 24-Hour Fitness, where she helped develop group exercise programs for instructors as well as conduct presentations and certifications throughout the United States. She teaches for 24-Hour Fitness in San Diego county and occasionally throughout California at special events. Page also holds certifications with both ACE and AFAA for group exercise and provides continuing education credits for ACE, AFAA, and PMA.

Page has developed five Pilates studios for California WOW Xperience fitness clubs in Thailand and South Korea and has trained more than 150 instructors at those clubs in the full mat and apparatus repertoire. Page was also a regional group exercise manager, managing five clubs in Thailand and three in Korea and overseeing nearly 1,000 group exercise classes per week.

She has starred in four videos with 24-Hour Fitness for group exercise instructors and was featured in Keli Roberts' *Pilates Quick Fix* video. She has also served as a fitness video technician for *Shape* magazine.

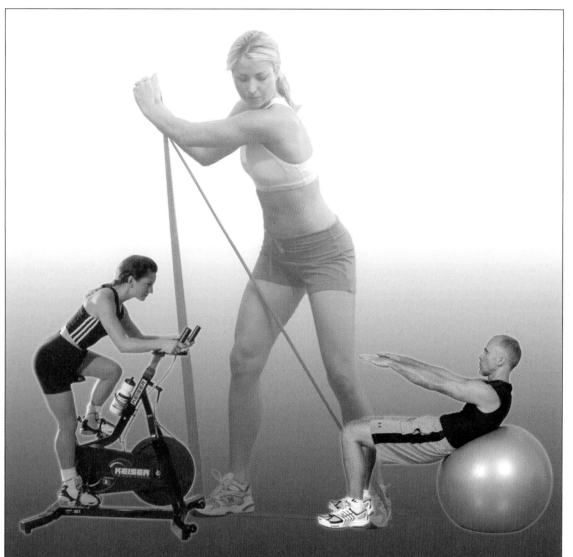

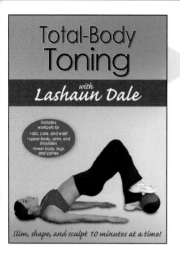
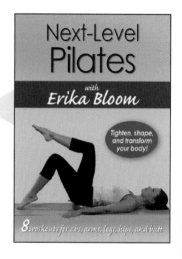
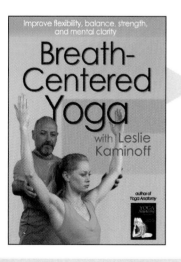
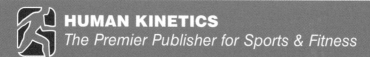